W0018423

Expressive Therapeutic Writing

This book brings engagement and conversation to a cross-pollination of creative and expressive writing and multi-modal art forms.

Through the lens of expressive arts therapy, the authors demonstrate how writing can reveal the unexpected that emerges from art making. The lineage of expressive arts therapy includes artful writing, poetry, associative, creative, and memoir, for example, to engage in self-discovery, growth, and restorative care. Each chapter is grounded in intermodal expressive arts with a central focus on creative and expressive writing, which is informed by movement, visual art, storytelling, music, sound, photography, and physical performance, including response art, and has writing prompts and invitations as well as playful and improvisational integrative arts writing explorations.

Creative arts therapists and expressive therapists actively searching for creative playful self-reflective writing practice will find this book a rewarding resource.

Krystal Leah Demaine, PhD, MT-BC, REAT, CTRS-C, RYT, music therapist, expressive arts therapist, and professor of expressive therapies at Endicott College, practices HEARTful healing note by note through song, story, poetry, and creative curiosity.

Tamar Reva Einstein, PhD, REAT, expressive arts therapist, poet/artist, and teacher, crosses cultural borders in Jerusalem with the arts as her mother tongue, threading writing and arts like her threaded beads and amulets.

Expressive Therapeutic Writing

Guiding Transformation and Restorative
Care through Intermodal Arts, Word
by Word

Krystal Leah Demaine
and Tamar Reva Einstein

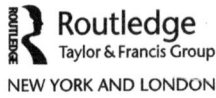

Routledge
Taylor & Francis Group

NEW YORK AND LONDON

Designed cover image: ©Getty

First published 2025
by Routledge
605 Third Avenue, New York, NY 10158

and by Routledge
4 Park Square, Milton Park, Abingdon, Oxon, OX14 4RN

Routledge is an imprint of the Taylor & Francis Group, an informa business

ISBN: 978-1-032-49019-9 (hbk)
ISBN: 978-1-032-49015-1 (pbk)
ISBN: 978-1-003-39187-6 (ebk)

DOI: 10.4324/9781003391876

Typeset in Times New Roman
by codeMantra

For our families.
Our parents and our sons.
With love.

Contents

About the Authors

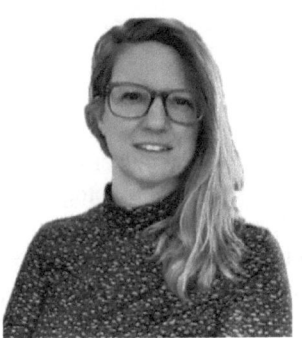

Krystal Leah Demaine, PhD, MT-BC, REAT, CTRS-C, RYT, is a professor of expressive therapies at Endicott College School of Visual and Performing Arts in Beverly, MA. She is a board-certified music therapist, registered expressive arts therapist, certified trauma and resilience specialist, certified in Trauma Sensitive HeartMath, and a registered yoga teacher. In her more than 20 years as an expressive arts clinician, writing has been used for sense-making through song, story, poetry, and creative reflection. Her book, *The Roots and Rhythm of the Heart: Our Musical Connection to Identity, Spirit, and Lineage* (2022), shares her story of grief, music, and HEARTful healing.

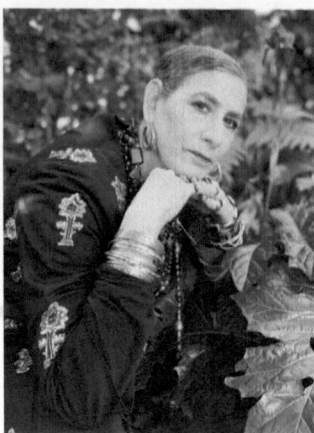

Tamar Reva Einstein, PhD, REAT, is a registered expressive arts therapist, who believes strongly that arts is her mother tongue. She has been writing since childhood; Tammy paints, dances, photographs, designs jewelry, and uses the creative, imagined, and transformative wisdom harvested from all of these to pass along to a new generation of creative arts therapists in Israel and the United States. She teaches, supervises, and practices, focusing on Jerusalem, crossing cultural borders with the arts as her passport and constant companion. Writing is a thread that has always connected the arts for her, similar to the string on which she threads her beads and amulets.

Foreword

… word by word invites you to write step by step, move by move. This last part of the book title tempted me to explore myself one word at a time—response: Write. Dare. Do it. And do it again.

This book is a practical guide without being too technical nor formalistic, yet also without following the idea that everything goes. The authors offer inspiring guidelines. Simple, yet not simplified as each invite leaves open space.

The two authors act as role models in an exemplary way. In that sense, writing is introduced on an eye-to-eye level with the reader, even though it is obvious that both speak up as expressive arts professionals in the clinical and educational realm.

Interestingly enough, they let the writing frames stand on their own in a non-judgmental and nonanalytical mode. They open the portal of writing, which includes prose, essays, poetry, memoirs, lists, letter writing, and notes based on an intermodal expressive arts context. Or, to use their words: *… we deeply believe in welcoming all to writing.* Literacy is an empowering gift.

We learn that writing may begin with orphaned books in languages we do not understand, with making words from other words, and with the blank page, the empty stage, the soothing sounds of pencils, and the improvisational playing with words, and writing may turn into a ritualistic practice, such as journaling, keeping a diary, a dream journal, or altering books. Writing can focus on hymns, praising common things, creating odes, prayers to ask for help, or in the sense of John O'Donohue, building a bridge between longing and belonging. The authors talk about "the spine of soulful writing."

The intermodal approach can include, to give some examples, writing in nature, and writing on stones, and can be also helpful to have a photograph or an artwork at hand and enter a process of ekphrastic writing. They introduce the value of metaphors in therapeutic writing, such as written self-portraits by developing a metaphor for the "self" like "self as a book," or "self as a flower," and show that figurative language can help clients to express their stories symbolically.

The poetic line of the Preface—*good poetry begins with a rose petal*—speaks poignantly about how they approach expressive therapeutic writing in the context of transformation and restorative care. They break it down in order to offer doable steps. And they withhold to undermine the impact of the written with proofs, such as case studies, or grades. They do the obvious thing: they speak for nobody else than themselves, their own experience, observations, and reflections. Their work is rooted in the phenomenological expressive arts approach. They consider writing as a gift and openly share their excitement and joy to work with writing in an intermodal way. We can observe that the art of writing stands on its own, an approach that follows Shaun McNiff's notion to validate the art as such, no matter its context. And which other modality—except visual arts and photography—is more sustainable than a piece of writing to which you can go back and reread any time?

This book offers endless intermodal writing frames, and I suggest going slow. It is a reference book you can use to receive an idea, or as a point of departure. Don't devour it, savor it.

I also need to mention the collaboration of the two authors. They mastered this challenging task in such a way that it reads as stemming from one author in terms of writing style, yet in terms of content, we hear two voices, each woman speaking up from her own unique experience. A true co-authoring that adds perspectives.

Having worked for more than 40 years in the field of expressive arts as faculty, psychotherapist, supervisor, and poet myself, I knew most of the frames, yet they succeeded in presenting each frame in a lively and fresh manner. This is actually the attitude to approach the exercises: the reader has the freedom to adapt in the way he/she needs it.

This book is for laypersons as well as for professionals; it addresses in its nonhierarchical mother tongue of the arts anybody interested in learning, exploring, receiving confirmation, guidelines, support, and inspiration.

I encourage you to approach this book with curiosity, for, as the authors remind us, curiosity includes a desire to know or learn to be inquisitive, meddlesome, and inquiring eagerly, as well as a desire to know or learn what is strange or unknown. Tammy and Krystal show the reader that to care for and to be curious are by its etymological roots connected. I do care for transformative writing, and I am curious to see where it continues to take us—my congratulations to this book.

Margo Fuchs Knill, PhD
Founding Dean
Division of Arts, Health and Society
European Graduate School
January 19, 2024

Preface

After David White

Good Poetry

Good poetry begins with
Not trying to write
A good poem
My beloved childhood writing teacher
Phillip Lopate
Used to read us
Grown-up poems
Or say: JUST WRITE!
And we did
Roberto, Xiomara, Lee…
And poems emerged in that New York City classroom
And were published
In our school
In the magazine called:
The Spicy Meatball
I was a monitor
I mimeographed
Turning the machine
Round
And round
And round
Inky hands
Waiting for the next class
Of writing
I always loved the words
Mine

Other's
Good poetry begins with
A soul that wants to speak
And when I invite
My adult students to write a poem
They are always surprised
And moved
To discover
What good poets they finally are
And we all agree
That poetry
Like its sister arts
It gets to the essence
Like those tons of rose petals needed to make a few ounces
Of essential rose oil
Good poetry
Begins with
A rose petal

—TRE Tamar Reva Einstein 2020

Acknowledgments

We acknowledge our parents and ancestors
who sparked our creativity and humanity
and a deep appreciation of peace and equality
and brought us into this world;
the ones who are alive and the ones who are no longer with us.
Our shared and non-shared mentors
who modeled arts
and imagination
as a mother tongue
Our beloved sons
who bring us joy and pride.
Our expressive arts therapy community
who supports, carries, and shares our journey as we move ahead.
To our students and supervisees
who teach us as much as we teach them.
To all of you, you know who you are,
who keep us grounded, playful, openhearted
and connected to our spiritual and cognitive roots.
fertilized by love
and composted by
ancient wisdom.

We give recognition to the following people who have contributed their time, wisdom, creativity, patience, and inspiration: Amanda Savage, Priya Sharma, Katya Porter, Teresa Fisher, Mitchell Kossak, Shaun McNiff, The Phabulous PhD Ladies, Michele Forinash, Cacky Mellor, Liza Hyatt, Barbara Black Koltuv, Christine Valters Paintner, Pat Allen, Donna Baier Stein, Phillip Lopate, Nancy Scherlong, and Margo Fuchs Knill and Paolo Knill.

Lastly, we would like to acknowledge each other for the unique and beautiful co-authoring experience that has deepened our love for one another and our love for words.

Thank you.
Krystal and Tamar

Introduction

Krystal Leah Demaine and Tamar Reva Einstein

Welcome

We invite you to enter the portal of writing. Come sit with us by our writing fire, as Shel Silverstein (1978) so poignantly mentions in his poem, *The Invitation* (p. 9). Crossing the threshold will be done through sound, movement, color, images, sensations, thoughts, and emotions. Here, you will experience what it means to be a creative human, a dabbler in the arts, a music appreciator, a craft enthusiast, a museum lover, and anyone who is tempted by or inspired by the ancient Greek muses of the arts and humanities, many connected to poetry: Calliope, Clio, Erato, Euterpe, Melpomene, Polyhymnia, Terpsichore, Thalia, and Urania. Each, in Greek mythology, represented and was a patron of all arts; specifically, in this book, they are the muses of writing as they entice you and welcome you into the mystical magical world of writing.

In this book, when we use the word *writing*, this includes prose, essays, poetry, memoirs, lists, letter writing, alphabetic letters, notes, writing in different languages, descriptive, autobiography, graffiti, tattooing, and any other way of writing that invites a person to express themselves. The door to writing awaits you; turn the handle when you are ready.

Writing in History

Writing is ancient and spans cultures and traditions. The origins of writing started with mark-making. People wanted and still want to leave their mark and use it to communicate their stories. In caves, and on stones worldwide, dots, slashes, and symbols have been found carved and painted on surfaces; this is believed to be the birth of writing. According to a recent online article in *Discover Magazine*, "Ancient humans' first written words are 20,000 years old," referring to the newest research findings on the history of writing, written in the *Cambridge Archeology Journal,* writing might have begun much earlier than priorly believed (Walters, 2023). The focus seemed to be on animals that they observed, and their mating and birthing seasons and cycles. This information, of

DOI: 10.4324/9781003391876-1

course, was extremely important to people who lived at that time as they were hunters and gatherers (Walters, 2023).

In our shared experience when people write they are still passionate about leaving their mark. One needs only look around to see that graffiti and street artists feel a need to publicly yet secretly write their special names, their tags, write pieces of poetry, political slogans, or inspiring quotes in very visible places. Posters at demonstrations, for example, can have a huge effect on people. Many of us are familiar with the ritual of carving things into trees, for example, the names of beloved people encircled with a heart. How about writing in bathroom stalls, what is that about? The toilet is not broken, the door is not broken, and things are left intact, yet people simply want to write messages and leave their mark in a place where other people will see it. We believe that writing, though very intimate, is also very powerful in relaying messages to the public.

Many of us know stories of children who have written in places they were not supposed to write. Perhaps this is a demonstration of power, but many children drew and wrote on walls, furniture, and clothing, leaving their mark. When you were a child, did you draw on the wall? When Tamar was a young child and left at home with an unliked babysitter, she went into her parents' room to fall asleep in their bed and ended up communicating her dissatisfaction with her parents' absence by drawing and writing all over her parents' orange velvet bedspread. In retrospect, while writing this book it seems that Tamar was marking and expressing her anger through that writing.

The power of writing is also very clear when one thinks about books that are banned or burned, or communities of people who are not allowed to relay their messages publicly in written form. Slave owners didn't understand that there was a whole language being communicated on quilts. A language within quilting and embroidering allowed black enslaved people in America to direct slaves to safety. The quilts were left out on clotheslines or windowsills of safe houses so that those who walked by their homes could see them. There was a secret code embedded within the quilt patterns and symbols that led folks to safety (Bryant, 2019). The history of writing is much wider and deeper than we can reach in this small section. Our bucket has been lowered into the deep well of writing history, but we invite you to continue to draw the history out at your own pace, within and beyond the pages of this book.

Structure of this Book

Now that you are sitting at the desk and before you dip your quill into the inkwell, we offer a compass to help direct you through the structure of the chapters that follow. Each chapter will begin with an abstract, which we call a welcome mat, to know what you are walking into. Each chapter will end with creative writing invitations, resources for further self-research, and the references that were mentioned within each chapter.

Resources will include recommended films, videos, websites, periodicals, museums, performance halls, exhibitions, artists' studios, libraries, books, poems, visual arts, meditations, recipes, songs, and other surprises.

Meet the Authors

The authors, who from this point on will be referred to as we or our, or by their first names, Tamar (a registered expressive arts therapist) and Krystal (a board-certified music therapist and registered expressive arts therapist), met during their doctoral studies at Lesley University in 2009. From then on, a close friendship developed which included, amongst other topics, our academic teaching. In shared conversations, we were surprised to discover how important writing had become to us both personally and in our teaching. Reflective writing, creative writing, poetry, and word invitations were shared from afar as we researched this common passion for penning. Simultaneously, we were aware that our immersion in multiple art languages enhanced and inspired us to write. Not necessarily academic writing, though that too has been a part of our lives. Like many who came before us, writing was not put on a separate pedestal but connected with other arts: Anais Nin, Isabelle Allende, Oliver Sacks, and Colette, for example, all engaged in multiple art forms and inspired our practices. We also want to take this opportunity to mention that we had very great models for maintaining engagement in more than one art form: Shaun McNiff, the late Lousie Montello, Mitchell Kossak, Suzanne Hanser, and the late Paolo Knill. How one creative art form fertilizes another is a gift; a garden of cacophonic sound, sights, and flavors might grow if tended to well. This is what we attempt to pass on to our students with our writing courses. Write from the heart, from the movement of your hands, from your associations, your memories; there is no right way as we write. Grammar, diction, and penmanship do not apply. We try to create a non-judgmental, contained, safe space in which past disheartening writing experiences can be transformed into new relationships with letters, words, sentences, and paragraphs. A world in which writing is therapeutic, inspirational, reflective, transformative, and cathartic.

The Authors First Exposure to Writing in Their Childhood

We have in common that we began writing at a very young age; we were very blessed to have been given the opportunity. We were those kids who continued to move their pens across the paper and still do as we write this book.

Both of us were gifted with writing programs as an integral part of our childhood education. In public school in New York City, in the 1960s, Tamar participated in a writing program taught by, among others, Phillip Lopate, created by the Teachers and Writers Collaborative, which originated from Herbert Kohl's idea to bring writers and artists into the public school system (Lopate, 1975). Tamar wrote poetry in those classes.

Tamar's poetry wiggled into other components of her life; from her master thesis and doctoral dissertation to her spiritual poetry writing in which she currently engages. In searching for some of her first-ever written poetry Tamar found the original handwritten and decorated copy of a poem written during her time at her childhood school, Public School 75, aptly named, The Emily Dickinson School. When Martin Luther King was murdered in 1968, Tamar's teachers discussed this in-depth in the multiracial and multicultural school. Tamar was seven years old. On the day the class commemorated the horrific killing, students were asked to write poems for a writing contest for the National Association for the Advancement of Colored People (NAACP) to honor and remember the reverend and black social activist. Tamar wrote a poem and was chosen as one of the winners of this contest. The words of the poem titled "Brotherhood" are:

> It will be a miracle when we see
> Different people living together peacefully
> People have tried, like Dr. Martin Luther King
> To open people's ears to hear freedom ring
> Animals live together, they don't even try
> But we treat others like they live in a pigsty
> Peacefulness is beautiful, why can't others see the light
> You should be treated equally whether you're Red, Black or White.

Tamar wrote the above poem when she was in elementary school; the content sadly is still current. As one of the contest winners, she and her family were in invited to attend an award ceremony at a special hall in Manhattan. It was almost impossible to contain her excitement, as Susan, the actor from the television show *Sesame Street*, handed Tamar a brass trophy of two hands shaking one another. A moment Tamar will never forget, which had such a big effect, that her doctoral studies were about multiculturalism and expressive arts therapy and included poetry writing. This serves as a reminder that our childhood writing can still stay relevant and that being raised in a world of expression through words crosses cultures until today. The writing mark was left on Tamar.

As a young girl in the 1980s, playing music, drawing pictures, writing stories, and short poems engaged Krystal in a way to communicate her young voice. A meaningful childhood memory was of her parents signing her up to participate in the "Kids to College" poetry and creative writing courses at age seven, held at the local community college.

As a child, Krystal wrote voraciously in her handwritten diaries. Generally, Krystal was introverted and shy and the journals gave her a place to tell her stories safely. She noted moments like her handmade Halloween costumes sewn by her mom and the time she chose purple balloons for her ninth birthday party which nine kids attended. She also wrote about being able to accompany her father to their penny candy and gift shop early in the morning as he prepared for customers. She organized the rock candy sticks, root beer barrels, Swedish fish, and colorful salt-water taffy in their large-mouthed glass jars. In an excerpt from December 1, 1986, when Krystal was nine, she described:

> Yesterday me and my dad went down on the Neck to work at the store. First, we went to get some strudel and hot choklat, but my dad got a coffee thow. Then we set up the store together. I organized the candy jars with my dad and then we started working. Then my mom and sister came for lunch. It was fun.

(The above excerpt is taken directly from Krystal's original childhood journal. The Neck refers to Bearskin Neck, an area of land located in Rockport, Massachusetts. Krystal's parents' gift shop, The Bearskin Neck Country Store, is still in business.)

As Krystal grew older, she began to integrate writing into other art forms that she became drawn to, specifically photography. She added reflective poems and stories in response to the photographic images she captured. Sometimes she took photos to match lyrics from her favorite songs. A glimmer of integrating the arts in her young years is a memory that Krystal holds dearly. In response to a photograph she took of a cherub statue in a small winter garden, Krystal wrote the following rhyming poem at the age of 13:

> Little white cherub you chipped your clay
> But you cheer up this garden on a dreary day
> So lonely you are among the weeds
> Grey days are here in a cold breeze
> You are all alone but not for a while
> I like your quiet smile and you have good style
> Make some new friends when springtime is here
> And flowers and greens grow more near
> Thank you cherub for your time
> You helped to remind me that things are just fine
>   — Krystal Demaine, 1991

Authors' Writing Process

This co-authored book was written through a ritual of weekly meetings; a shared routine that included conversing, writing, imagining, remembering, typing, and exploring how writing has been a part of our creative practices as expressive arts therapists for over three decades. This first step of creative improvised writing seemed to fit the space in which it occurred; two kitchens that were chosen as our writing places in our respective homes, thousands of miles apart. The conjuring of the words is so similar to the improvisational skills of well-seasoned chefs. Words and stories were shared, told aloud, like family recipes, then expanded upon, and whole verbal meals were prepared online via Zoom with a seven-hour time zone difference. Krystal was cooking breakfast while Tamar was making dinner. As co-authors, we worked together and harvested our writing experiences; we refined and filtered our narrative until we got to the essence of the writing. Like a reduced sauce, our writing in our kitchens became more concentrated, thicker, and hopefully more flavorful for readers.

Co-creating in all of the arts, for example, music, dance, visual arts, photography, drama, and singing, is a process that enhances and amplifies collaboration. We experienced this in our process of writing this book. Writing can be a very lonely and somewhat isolating art form. Writers have said how lonely it is to sit in a room and write. Co-authoring softened and dissolved any form of isolation in our writing. A wonderful example of how isolation can be used for cathartic and healing writing has been created by Suleika Jaouad (2023) in her online platform, *The Isolation Journals*, which chronicles her journey through her most recent bout with cancer. On the banner of the website homepage in big letters, with a background from a painting that she painted, states, "Transforming isolation into creative solitude and connection." Jaouad continues and writes, "The Isolation journals were founded on the idea that life's interruptions are invitations to deepen our creative process" (Jaouad, 2023, para 1). She and her husband, famed musician Jon Batiste, have recently released a documentary film, *American Symphony*, that illustrates this poignantly and artfully (Heineman, 2023).

The experience we shared in writing this book was reciprocal and collaborative in every way. Meeting weekly and sometimes daily invited creative exchange for cultivating the richness of our art, therapy, teaching, and parenting. The co-creating made the writing process much less lonely; it was fun and at times brought us to tears both in joy and sorrow.

Why We Are Writing this Book

The seed of writing this book was planted when we exchanged thoughts and ideas for writing courses that Krystal was creating at Endicott College and Tamar had been teaching at a phototherapy institute for over 20 years in Jerusalem. As the years went by and we continued to collaborate and cross-pollinate we discovered that writing was a thread that wove together and deepened many of our students' artmaking experiences. Thread by thread, word by word, an imaginary loom was used to intertwine and make sense as the word weavers, connected, wrote, and shared what they had crafted.

We both teach courses and lead workshops at universities, conferences, and in other communities globally including nurse training programs, with psychologists, artists, and educators, in juvenile probation, hospice care, acute care centers, schools and their staff, forensic psychiatry, addiction treatment facilities, the public welfare realm, special education, and trauma centers. Both of us also work as clinicians and supervisors. We have used writing in all of these settings.

Now comes the magic! Students and participants have repeatedly told us stories of how completely caught off guard and surprised they were as to how writing allowed them to express, create, expose, transform, and empower: it felt as if each letter was part of an alchemy of writing. It is astounding to us as we witness our students' and participants' experiences and feel a calling to share some of these stories within this book. We find it enchanting to be present in the transformation as it gets to the heart of our participants' writing, and their emotional, spiritual, creative, challenged, and precious lives.

Rather than make writing a chore, we find, for instance, that many of our students enjoy writing academic reflective essays; and have asked to write beyond the maximum page requirements, adding in personal narratives and cathartic moments that happened while writing and looking over their semester journals. Reflective writing allows students to make sense of the whole semester. Such self-contemplative writing is authentic and deliberate; it comes from the heart; it is somatic from the body; it allows an opportunity to extract the inner thoughts and invites a way of sifting through the sand of the personal narrative. Writing is an art language and when we begin to generate expressive writing it promotes deeper understanding. Writing gets to the depths of the soul and sometimes it surprises people how quickly writing taps into those depths. It seems that in each of us, there is a well that is often untapped brimming with words and stories waiting to be drawn out.

The Gift of Writing

As we have mentioned, writing has incredible possibilities for transformation. We are not saying that writing is the best way to heal or the most profound form of creativity; we are saying that writing is a powerful way to express oneself from our experiences. Writing can be created alongside and interwoven with dancing, painting, music-making, artmaking, photography, and many other art forms. As writer Kurt Vonnegut (2006) suggested, no matter what art form one engages in, the arts allow one to become more aware of the inner self and soul. Writing is a gift in the sense that one can always go back to it, even from decades before to revisit one's deepest and most private inquiries and stories. For example, Dr. Ruth, a noted sex therapist, at the age of 95 years old during the COVID-19 lockdown re-read her childhood journals (some written during the Holocaust) and decided to focus her attention on loneliness (Gilbert, 2023). Dr. Ruth's experience gives us an example of how rereading things we have written in the past can open the doors of our memories and emotions to new unresearched parts of ourselves. Transformation is always possible at any stage of life through writing; it's the gift that keeps giving. Writing is a form of alchemy that as Gass (2010) wrote can, "change the world into words" (p. 37).

Resources

Places to Visit

Authors Ridge at Sleepy Hollow Cemetery, 248 Bedford Street, Concord MA.

Within Sleepy Hollow Cemetery, there is an area known as Authors Ridge where several classic authors are buried, including Henry David Thoreau, Louisa May Alcott, and Ralph Waldo Emerson.

Programs to Explore

Kids to College Programs

Check your local community college summer listings to see if a Kids to College Program is offered. This could give your child, who may be an early bloomer, a leg up on a field that might inspire them.

Videos to Watch

"How a Group of Women in This Small Alabama Town Perfected the Art of Quilting" is narrated beautifully and produced by *The New York Times*. This November 18, 2018, video found on their YouTube channel shares the story of quilt codes made by Black Enslaved people in America in the 1830s, which helped bring them to safe places. This singing alone will stir you; we guarantee it! https://www.youtube.com/watch?app=desktop&v=YHEqYVzSs7U

This November 13, 2023, interview from *Eyewitness News ABC7NY* with Dr. Ruth shares what she refers to as the new epidemic in the world: loneliness. It is found on the ABC7NY YouTube channel:

https://youtube.com/watch?v=srD3GkjPHZ8&si=HVNlw95gGgVLga44.

Websites to Explore

Banksy Official Website https://www.banksy.co.uk/

The official website for the world-infamous graffiti artist known as Banksy.

References

Bryant, M.C. (2019, May 3). Underground railroad quilt codes: What we know, what we believe, and what inspires us. *Smithsonian Center for Folklife and Cultural Heritage*. https://folklife.si.edu/magazine/underground-railroad-quilt-codes

Gass, W.H. (2010). *A temple of texts*. Knopf Doubleday Publishing Group.

Gilbert, G. (2023, November 9). Dr. Ruth saved people's sex lives. Now she wants to cure loneliness. *New York Times.* https://www.nytimes.com/2023/11/09/nyregion/dr-ruth-loneliness-ambassador.html

Heineman, M. (Director) (2023). *American symphony.* [Film, streaming]. Netflix; Our Time Projects, Mercury Studios, Higher Ground Productions.

Jaouad, S. (2023). *Transforming life's interruptions into creative grist.* The Isolation Journals. https://www.theisolationjournals.com/

Lopate, P. (1975). *Being with children.* Doubleday.

Silverstein, S. (1978). *Where the sidewalk ends.* HarperCollins Children's Books.

Vonnegut, K. (2006, November 5). Letter to Xavier High School. https://news.lettersofnote.com/p/make-your-soul-grow

Walters, S. (2023, April 20). Ancient humans first written words are 20,000 years old. *Discover Magazine.* https://www.discovermagazine.com/the-sciences/ancient-humans-first-written-words-are-20-000-years-old

Chapter 1

Intermodal Arts and Writing
How One Art Fertilizes the Other

Krystal Leah Demaine and Tamar Reva Einstein

Welcome Mat: This chapter will share the authors' backgrounds and personal stories that illuminate their choice to write this book together, including how the thread of writing has woven its way through their creative practices as expressive arts therapists intertwined with music, dance, and visual arts in higher educational settings, experiential workshops, clinical practice, and in their own self-reflective and artistic writing endeavors and explorations. The cross-pollination of the arts has been beautifully described by Anais Nin (1981), "each art must nourish the other" (p. 264).

The Arts as our Mother Tongue

As clinicians, we come from the world of expressive arts therapy, in which different words have been used to describe the process of using the arts together in therapy. We want to explore specific terms we were taught and continue using in our work. These terms can be applied to non-therapeutic work as well. Even psychologist Abraham Maslow noticed, "A musician must make music, an artist must paint, a poet must write if he is to be ultimately at peace with himself. What a man can be, he must be" (1954, p. 93). We will be focusing on intermodal expressive arts, intermodal transfer, integrated arts, and aesthetic feedback. To clarify, when we write the term *arts*, we are referring to different art forms, for example: music, movement, singing, choreography, wordplay, dance, narrative, poetry, photography, sound-making, sculpture, digital arts, painting, drawing, drama, writing, and all forms of creative or imaginary play.

As Knill described the practice of expressive arts therapy in the film *A Time to Dance: The Life and Work of Normal Canner*, "It is becoming masterful in moving between the arts" (Brownwell & Wilcoxen, 1998, 0:41:49). When the profession of expressive arts therapy was born at Lesley College (now University) in the 1970s, under the direction of Shaun McNiff, Paolo Knill, Norma Canner, and colleagues, the concept of moving between the arts was the cornerstone of everything that was taught and learned. Flowing between the arts was a new therapeutic language that expressive arts therapy graduate students

DOI: 10.4324/9781003391876-2

were all taught to speak fluently. This fluency was and is sometimes confounding to other helping professionals, who sometimes refer to the expressive arts therapist as a "Jack of all trades." Of course, the continuation of that phrase, as written by Shakespeare, is "master of none, but oftentimes better than a master of some" (Van Es, 2010). Knill wrote, simply and clearly, "Imagination is intermodal" (Knill, Barba, Fuchs, 1995, p. 25). When we imagine, all of our senses are awake, when we create from this imagination, all of our senses are also awake. So, it makes sense that in expressive arts therapy, intermodality is our mother tongue.

Intermodality and Intermodal Arts Transfer

The term intermodal arts in essence means to move from one art form to the other. A concept rich in the aforementioned Lesley University expressive arts therapy history, intermodality is the essential key to practicing as an expressive arts therapist.

When Krystal introduces intermodality to her undergraduate students, she invites each person to bring a meaningful personal photograph. The students place their photographs face down on a mat in the middle of the floor without precise directives. After asking permission to touch the photos, Krystal turns each photo face up and asks for a certain number of students to volunteer to use their imagination and make up 30-second spoken storytelling of the image. After a few of the imaginative stories are shared the group along with Krystal collectively exclaims out loud, "**What's the real story?!!**" The owner of the image then shares their authentic photo story.

Once all of the stories are shared by those who choose to share, the group works together to think about the order of the photos as if they were a visual choreography determining which image starts, ends, and is in the middle. At this point in the process, students are invited to move the photos around until the entire group agrees that they have reached a moment that feels like the best sequence for the story. Once the visual choreography is set the mode of sound is added: in other words, the photographic dance receives a film score. The group collaborates to determine a sound that each photograph evokes. The sounds are projected aurally, created by the students' voices and bodies, as Krystal points to each photo one by one. Next, the participants are invited to move as inspired by the photos while making the sound. At this point, they become a dance company and a choir.

The peak of the entire experience culminates with the creation of a moving human fluid sculpture. It is important to mention that this sculpture is rendered and performed repeatedly until it becomes completed in the eyes and bodies of all participants. The completeness is felt when the group agrees they have brought their sculpture to its full expression. This exemplifies both intermodal artwork and intermodal expressive arts transfers.

What began as a one-dimensional photographed image becomes a multi-dimensional, choreographed movement experience with a personal soundtrack created by the participants, who are asked to write in their journals about the entire process and product. The writing allows students to digest their understanding of intermodal expressive arts and reframes that a very personal photograph becomes part of an ensemble. After writing in their journals the students sit in a large circle and as a group share thoughts, feelings, and emotions that were written about the experience.

Integrated Arts

Our understanding of the term integrated arts is that all of the arts are connected; and that no art form exists without the other. We believe that the arts work together and not as sole entities. For example, when we play music, we intrinsically move the body as we play our instrument and sing our songs, which can contain a story within the lyrics and a dance from the movement. A starting point for the arts may begin with movement, which comes from anywhere in the body. The movement can be subtle such as breathing, or big with large jumps and leaps, or silent and internal like neurons firing and the heart beating. When we paint or sculpt, write, dance, play, sing, or act we inherently move our body part by part or perhaps all together. Importantly though, all of the arts are joined in an undercurrent by the glue of creativity, play, flow, and imagination. Tamar has a strong memory from her expressive art therapy graduate studies, over decades ago, with her mentor, Shaun McNiff whom she recalled emphasizing that, *all arts start with movement, they start with the body*. We interpret this statement as any bodily experience. McNiff who has served as a mentor to us both has influenced our artmaking, clinical work, teaching, and supervising. Through his guidance and our collective experiences, we translate intermodal arts and integrated arts as the soul, psyche, and spirit speaking through all of the arts both in an intermodal and an integrative language, wherein the arts are our mother tongue.

In the classroom, the workshop, or the group therapy session there is no audience. Rather, the students or participants are a group of witnesses serving as a container and holders of the space for each person to have a deep arts conversation with what they have created.

In both theories (intermodal expressive arts and integrated arts), art is the mother tongue and it needs no explanation or interpretation. This means that we use the arts to communicate the emotion, the felt sense, and the feeling. Arts invigorate us, give us tingles, provoke movement, and conjure thoughts and emotions. We don't need to explain ourselves when we can express our internal experiences through the arts. No matter which theory we focus on, the intermodal or the integrated arts, something that is shared is that moving between the arts and intertwining the arts amplifies and clarifies the meanings, emotions, and thought processes of the creator of the piece. As earlier mentioned in the example from Krystal's classroom, the students communicated a deeper understanding and expression of a photo by adding sound, movement, and performance until they felt a sense of completeness through their expression. The addition or integration of each art form allows for a greater personal expression for the client, student, or participant engaged in the experience.

Written Aesthetic Feedback

Aesthetic response, artistic response, response art, and artistic feedback are all indigenous terms to the field of expressive arts therapy. To reference the seminal book from our field, *Minstrels of the Soul: Intermodal Expressive Therapy*, the aesthetic response was described as "A distinct *response,* with a bodily origin to an occurrence in the imagination, to an artistic act, or the perception of an artwork" (Knill, Barba, Fuchs, 1995, p. 71). Within this book, we choose to address the concept of written aesthetic feedback. When we use writing, in all of its forms, we honor and interweave words to and with other arts.

Knill, Barba, Fuchs (1995) describe the felt sense, relating to Gendlin's (1978) work in the 1970s on focusing. A felt sense indicates the sensations one experiences when creating an image. Aesthetic experiences stir sensations in our body, perhaps give us chills, spark emotions, invoke a desire to move, and awaken a strong drive to create; paint, write, make sounds, say words, play, dance, sing, or express in other art forms. In daily language, we use terminology that refers to these experiences such as saying, *I was so moved by that painting, that piece of music gave me goosebumps,* or *the poem brought me to tears.* Sometimes we are stopped short by art, we become speechless, and our bodies do not need words at times like that. Such physical expressions communicate the bodily sensations or the connection between the soul and the senses evoked by the power of the arts.

When Tamar was a graduate student at what was then Lesley College, between 1985 and 1987, she found herself writing poems as feedback to fellow students in group supervision and to clients at one of her clinical practicum sites, a therapeutic clinic for homeless people in Cambridge staffed by an interdisciplinary team. This writing of poems was completely unplanned and took her by surprise. Tamar had never responded person to person with a poem until that moment. It began at first in the well-contained, professional, and arts-based supervision. She would watch, listen, witness, and feel the student presenting, and words would flow out in metaphoric poems. When she shared the first one aloud, the echoes and resonance from the student presenter and the group leader, Paolo Knill, as well as from the other students, were powerful. The poem had gone right to the essence, in metaphor.

While the student was presenting, Tamar watched the student talk about how overwhelmed she was as she walked around the inner circumference of the circle; within which the students and Paolo sat on the floor of the Carriage House.

The student spoke faster, walked faster, and began running in dizzying circles as she said aloud what she had been doing with her first clients and how it made her feel. When the student finally sat back down in her empty spot, she was sweating, crying, and exhausted both physically and emotionally. The group was given time to create aesthetic responses, and so was she. Tamar looked at the woman, and felt so moved; as if she had just witnessed a sacred ritual. A transformative rite of passage. In moments Tamar's pen moved quickly across the page, almost as quickly as the student's running, as a poem emerged about how airplanes fly so quickly that the sonic boom we hear is a little bit after they pass us by; traveling faster than the speed of sound. Tamar experienced the student as becoming such a winged plane, moving faster than she could hear herself. In discussion, during the sharing time, the student spoke about how she recognized a pattern in her life of moving too fast, of needing to slow down, and that she was not aware of the sonic booms she was causing. Paolo, who was among many things, a physicist, loved the metaphor.

Tamar began writing these feedback poems to each student in supervision; and then dared to write feedback poems at her clinical internship, referred to as practicum. One example of aesthetic feedback in an internship setting occurred before one-on-one supervision. One day at the homeless clinic, after working with a woman who was a former English literature professor with a severe mental illness that rendered her homeless woman, Tamar sat alone and looked at the watercolor the woman had painted that day. She painted different shapes in blues, greens, and ochres, that reminded her of a mountainous view. Tamar wrote the expected progress notes, and then a poem about the painting. Tamar then shared the poem with her site supervisor. The supervisor was emotionally moved. Tamar and her supervisor discussed that perhaps, given that the client was a literature buff, often speaking about poets, for example, Sylvia Plath, Tamar could ask her if she wanted to hear the poem. The next time Tamar met with the woman, she asked and the woman did want to hear the reflective poem that she wrote. Tamar read it and the woman was very surprised that Tamar had taken time to do such a thing, and reported she felt some clarity through the words. Tamar continued to write poems about her work when she came to art therapy, which was sporadic due to the client being mentally ill and homeless. Tamar's master's thesis topic became clear; she wrote about metaphoric poetry writing in expressive arts therapy.

In 2009, Tamar returned to Lesley University to begin her doctoral work on multiculturalism and the expressive arts therapies in Jerusalem, based on her work on both sides of this overlapping, conflicted, and beautiful city with the expressive arts as her passport. As the doctorate emerged, Tamar found herself moving between academic writing, painting, sewing, dancing, and yes, once again, metaphoric response poems. All of the art forms were included in her arts-based research dissertation, "Sew it Seams." Tamar was home again. The following poem was written in response to an hour-long interview with one of her dissertation research participants, who said the words, "sisterhood of suffering." The words left a deep imprint on Tamar who was moved to spontaneously create a very large painting and then write a poem to the painting. The poem was originally printed in red.

The Sisterhood of Suffering

From within
the wallpapered womb
of the sisterhood of suffering,
Women wail,
Women chant,
Women pray,
Women beg,
Women cry out,
In pain,
Lamenting the loss
of their connecting,
communal blood.
From within
the wallpapered womb
of the sisterhood of suffering,
this red garbed sorority
seeks placental peace.

Response Art in Therapy and Education

Although this book is focused on writing, we cannot only refer to written aesthetic responses and feel strongly that all response art needs to be addressed. An expert on aesthetic response and artistic response, Barbara Fish (2019), referred to the practice of response art; and researched and identified how four important and highly regarded art therapists define response art as the following: "The practice of response art is referred to: 'visual empathetic response' (Franklin, 1990, p. 44), 'responsive art making' (Moon, 1999, p. 78), 'visual empathy' (Ramseyer, 1990, p. 118), and 'art for professional self-processing' (Wadeson, 2003, p. 208)" (p. 122).

For expressive arts therapists, it is relevant to respond to a client's art through art; this is response art. The art could come in any form as noted above and is not limited to visual or written forms. Franklin (2010) wrote, "With careful attunement, art therapists can develop unique, aesthetic forms of empathetic resonance. This territory presents significant opportunities for the artist within the art therapist to be active and of service to others" (p. 166). In addition, Nash (2020) stated,

A common theme found in the literature review is the capacity of response art to hold and contain complex, confusing, or unsettling feelings aroused in the work. Also creating artworks make internal phenomenon available for further work through the viewing and sharing with others, particularly one's supervisor, to work with partially processed material, to understand the therapist's countertransference reactions and experiences, and to build empathy.

(p. 9)

Careful paying attention to how the therapist feels and is left affected by one's clients or students can be deciphered and expressed in the language of the arts; in supervision as well as in the therapist's therapy.

Krystal has experienced such conscious and unconscious emotional responses to her student's works at times. An example of a written aesthetic response from Krystal's music therapy course is when students respond in written reflection to each other after they create a musical life review (Demaine, 2022). The musical life review is an autobiographical chronological soundtrack that they share, and then write a five-page reflective essay about this musical memoir. In the class, each student tells their story with their musical life review soundtrack playing in the background. The other students are given oil pastels, pens, and paper and asked to write a soulful, authentic, and respectful response, reflection, association, or reaction to the storyteller. This is not about giving a critique, but rather communicating to the student how their story and soundtrack affected the student witnesses. The closing ritual of this exercise is that each presenter is gifted with the responses from all of their classmates and Krystal. Krystal has noticed that it is often hard for people to hold off in reading their responses, they want to read them as quickly as possible. It is impossible to corral their curiosity; which leads us to remember how important it is for people to receive non-judgmental supportive and artistic feedback, in all aspects of our profession including in supervision, therapy, and self-care/self-reflection. The responses are kept by the students which allows them to revisit at home and for years to come.

The Importance of Words in Expressive Arts Groups

Humans use words to make meaning and express emotions, thoughts, and feelings. We are the only mammals that communicate through verbal language that can be understood among others; at least as far as we know. We need words to make sense of our experiences. There is a beautiful and strong verbal aspect in the expressive arts therapies, as if communication through words is an art form of its own. This speaks to those who refer to expressive therapies as a non-verbal form of therapy. No matter which modality we are immersed in as a therapist, client, or participant we often end up using words to get to the essence at the end of the experience. This is not to say that sharing verbally or through words exclusively occurs after or during a therapy session; words and language can occur at any time and in diverse ways, including while people are creating. There can be a moment in a therapy session when someone can look at the piece of art they have made and through conversation clarity is thusly brought to the experience. We are not saying that writing, dance, music, or any of the arts replace words, we are saying that words work as a magnifying glass in the process of clarifying human experiences. Writing things down is also a very powerful tool of documentation and something you can go back to. When one writes something down it often gives a deeper understanding of thoughts, feelings, and emotions.

In a non-therapeutic group that meets once a week to address the chaotic emotions that have arisen during the 2023 war between Hamas and Israel, a participant was quietly writing in her journal while viewing her three-dimensional collage made of ripped papers. Surprisingly she wanted to share her writing which was not her usual mode of communication; she usually did not want to share her writing, but this time she immediately exclaimed aloud, "*I want to read what I wrote!*" She shared words that had become a poem and when she got to the word *pyre*, she began sobbing. Tamar put a hand on the participant's shoulder and invited her to continue writing as her tears flowed down her face. After the other participants gave her feedback the participant shared that she had found the writing to be cathartic and felt less heavy than when she arrived in the group. Tamar invites people to take photographs of their work or take their work home and continue the artmaking process if they choose.

A few days later the participant shared photographs of the peak of the cathartic experience which was that she actually burned the piece of three-dimensional art, alone, and on her own accord, and then felt that she had let go of the heavy emotions and feelings that she was holding in her body. Writing about the art was what allowed her to engage and begin this cathartic process.

It is important to note the intermodal process here, the participant transferred from collage to writing, to burning, and then more writing. It was the writing that served as the anchor and pinpointed the meaning of the emotions and feelings.

Another example of an intermodal process tethered in writing was in a group of 40 seasoned educational psychologists who participated in professional development training. Tamar integrated writing tasks alongside phototherapy and arts-based invitations. The participants asked if they needed to share their writing within the large group. Tamar replied that sharing was welcome if the writers felt comfortable sharing aloud. They found it very intimidating if not impossible to openly read what they had written which led to a very wonderful discussion about disclosure in therapy. As therapists, we ask our clients to share information and disclose what is happening in their lives verbally out loud regularly, but when we are asked to share ourselves, we realize the challenges involved in this task. Isn't it ironic that professionals who expect that their clients will open up and share with them freely have difficulty opening up and disclosing their personal experiences in art or writing? Sharing has to do with trust building. These psychologists were asked to take photos and continue to write about the images they captured through their photos on an everyday basis for the next two months to become acquainted with and more comfortable with writing and sharing the intimacy that writing expresses and exposes. Tamar explained before leaving the psychologists that the word *overexposure* is actually from the world of photography from the darkroom; there is a difference between overexposure and exposure. The psychologists were afraid of overexposure.

Noting the Field of Bibliotherapy and Poetry Therapy

We use writing as one of the arts modalities in our work as expressive arts therapists. We need to note that neither of us is trained or certified as bibliotherapists or poetry therapists, and we do want to mention and honor those fields, as the book is about writing and transformation. One can be professionally trained as a bibliotherapist or poetry therapist. According to the International Federation for Biblio-Poetry Therapy website (2023), "The terms poetry therapy, applied poetry facilitation, journal therapy, bibliotherapy, Biblio/poetry therapy, and poetry/journal therapy are all intended to reflect the interactive use of literature and/or writing to promote growth and healing" (para 1). We love writing and spreading that love to our students, clients, and participants in many ways. This is often interwoven with other arts. It conjures for both of us our childhood memories of Charlotte the spider, in the book *Charlotte's Web*, who literally wove words, and knew their innate power (White & Williams, 1952).

Welcoming Everyone to Write

As clinicians, artists, and group leaders, we deeply believe in welcoming all to writing. Working on two sides of the world does not change this belief, but certainly does invite us to diversely different aspects of welcoming. Beverly, Massachusetts, USA, and Jerusalem, Israel, are quite different.

From Krystal's perspective welcoming everyone to write includes finding a shared safe space in which everyone's opinions, ideas, feelings, genders, origins, religious and spiritual beliefs, clothing and body adornment, races, abilities, age, socio-economic status, and life experience are warmly embraced and fortified. Being authentic and writing from the many genuine parts of what makes them human. This is assumed but also said out loud, at the first meeting, that reciprocal respect and honor of the people, the material, the process and product, and the space are an integral part of expressive arts therapy training and how they will contribute to the world.

From Tamar's perspective in working in Jerusalem, as it pertains to writing, welcoming is made of the same materials that Krystal creates but has the added ingredient of geopolitical conflict. When we incorporate writing in groups, we encourage writing in one's mother tongue, and for Tamar that includes Arabic, and then reading out loud the piece first in the mother tongue and then in the language that the majority of the group understands. We both want our groups to hear the sound, the song, and the accent of the language in which it has been written. We also strongly believe that writers feel more included when they are invited to write in their first language even if it takes more time in the group to translate the piece. Tamar believes that taking time to translate deepens the understanding of the piece to everyone, including the writer. This knowledge is partially due to Tamar's personal experience of speaking more than one language; English, Hebrew, and Arabic, but writing always in her mother tongue: English.

Alongside the term mother tongue are two other connected concepts that are directly related to the speaking aloud of the written word; the reason mother tongue is chosen for writing may be caused by these words: prosody and motherease (fatherease/parentease). Prosody refers to the melodic sense of speech which gives inflection, contour, and thus meaning to verbal utterances (Hirst, 2005). When a baby is born, and sometimes in utero, caregivers speak in a sing-songy manner referred to as motherease where vocal tonality increases as does the pitch and words are spoken in a lilting manner; at just 18 weeks the fetus can detect sounds (Woodward, 2019). Furthermore, a systematic review of the fetal understanding of the maternal voice conducted by Carvalho et al. (2019) identified that newborns and end-of-gestation fetuses were able to react and discriminate the maternal compared to other female voices. The results were based on the fetal reaction of neural and cardiac activity, and the baby's motor response through increased sucking and head-turning. Some people grow up in homes that are bi-, tri-, or multilingual where the "mother tongue" may be chosen by an individual they are living with and not by the individual themselves.

The Gift of Literacy: Cultivating Writing for Everyone

From time to time, we work with groups of people who do not know how to write or were never allowed to learn how to write, which is referred to as analphabetic, rendering such people, often women, completely illiterate. In fact, in 2015, *The Guardian* reported the United Nations found that among the world's illiterate population, two-thirds of those are women aged 15 years and above (Ford, 2015). Writing in some cultures was and still is unacceptable, prohibited, or even forbidden for women. In some cultures, prohibitive writing is a way to control and limit the expression and receiving of information. There are many places in which the therapist is the conduit, the translator, or the scribe and is relied upon to transcribe spoken word into lyric or poem or perhaps a drawing or physical movement into a written story or narrative.

Sometimes people have physical, neurological, developmental, emotional, and/or cognitive challenges or other hurdles that hinder the physicality of writing. Still, they want a written story so the therapist or another participant becomes the scribe. For example, for teachers of young children, there is a familiar practice of allowing a student to contribute to the group by the teacher writing for them. In many of Krystal's groups with young children, the story or song is often transcribed by an adult while the child shares their words that contribute to the arts-based expressions. For her clients with intellectual disabilities, drawing or musical instrument sounds sometimes serve as a replacement for spoken verbal language.

In Tamar's private practice, a visually impaired client created three-dimensional plasticine figures and shapes and then wrote free-flowing stories and associative writing in Braille. She brought the brailler, a machine that writes in braille, to her session; she wrote, and then read aloud. The therapy became a ritual of weekly storytelling and story writing based on the three-dimensional plasticine figures that the client created. Tamar then transcribed her client's words with pen and paper as they were spoken.

Toward the completion of therapy, the client admitted that she had never thought of writing as a way to just let loose and get her story out. The client's professional work was listening to English-spoken movies and writing the Hebrew subtitles on a special computer. So, for the client, writing was work and it was very perfection-oriented. The writing experience in therapy opened up a whole new world for her to continue writing about her past personal and life-changing traumas, and her future dreams, and allowed her to move on in life.

It is important to note that the movement or intermodal transfer between the kneading, molding, and shaping of the plasticine to the writing was what built sense-making and emotional clarity in the sessions. In this instance, writing and reading aloud was an affirming experience.

Writing Invitations

1 **Welcoming and Releasing the Day**

When you wake up in the morning, before you do anything else, even while still in your bed, take a photograph to welcome the day. Later on in the day, take a moment to write one sentence about this photograph. In the evening before you go to sleep, take a photograph to say goodbye to the day and write a few words about it either at that moment or the next morning. Do this for at least a month. When you look back at the writing cycle see if you find meaningful moments that you can reread and perhaps you might want to continue this practice again or in cycles.

2 **Orphaned Books in Languages We Do Not Understand**

Find a book in a language that you do not understand. Perhaps this is an orphaned book, one that someone is no longer using, on the street, outside of the library being given away, or a book you feel you no longer need. Look at the book carefully, look at the shape of the letters, and the direction in which the letters are written. Is it up and down, left to right, do you understand the direction in which it is meant to be read? Now, sit down, and imagine what is written in this book and write it down. Keep looking up at different pages, especially if there are any illustrations, to get some input on adding details to what you are writing. Imagine the person who orphaned this book and why they didn't want it anymore. Why didn't they want this book anymore? You can write over the other letters in the book, write on the blank pages. Give the book a new title and make it your own. Decorate and re-make the cover. Then do some reflective writing about how it made you feel to explore this book. Did it connect you to your language, to your origins, to stories you have heard? Is there someone to whom you'd like to share this book and show it.

3   **Making Words from Other Words**

Write the word **WELCOME** at the top of a blank page. Use each letter to think of all the words you can write that begin with that letter. This will leave you with a list of words. This list of words begins with each letter of your name. You will have a W list, an E list, an L list, a C list, an O list, an M list, and another E list. Take a few moments to look at your list and circle words that seem meaningful to you at the moment. In other words, they can be attractive, repulsive, curiosity-building, interesting, mysterious, surprising, and/or inviting. Once circled, take those words and use them to write anything: a short story, a poem, a list of questions, a letter, or anything else. Take a break: a few minutes, a few days, or a month; the time frame depends on your needs and capabilities. Allow enough time to deeply absorb these words. Go back to this piece later on, and reread it, and give it a title. See if a theme has arisen that you did not notice before. If you are so moved, you may want to create art in response to this. Photographs, collages, paintings, music, songs, sculptures, or perhaps a dance. You might even be inspired to cook or make a nature-based assemblage. Write about this too!

Resources

Books to Explore

The Little Prince (1943) by Antoine de Saint-Exupéry, published by Harcourt Brace & Co.

The Little Prince is one of our go-to books for sharing with our students when discussing the concept of looking at things from a new perspective.

Tharp, T. (2003). *The creative habit: Learn it and use it for life.* Simon & Schuster.

The Creative Habit written by dance choreographer Twyla Tharp offers wonderful first-hand insight to get the art in the groove of creating.

Upaya Center: Natalie Goldberg Writing Lectures, https://www.upaya.org/person/natalie-goldberg/

The Upaya Center offers a variety of Buddhist-centered workshops both online and in person at their physical location in Santa Fe, New Mexico, USA. We have attended amazing writing workshops with writer Natalie Goldberg, who teaches writing workshops at the center regularly. You can learn more about Natalie Goldberg by visiting her website https://nataliegoldberg.com/.

Interviews

In this filmed interview with William Kentridge, he shows and discusses his journey over decades of being told he had to choose between art forms, feeling like a failure, and then owning that he was a multifaceted ARTIST. You can watch the video titled, 'William Kentridge Interview: How We Make Sense of the World', on YouTube on the Louisiana Channel: https://www.youtube.com/watch?v=G11wOmxoJ6U. It was uploaded on October 1, 2014.

Films

Norma Canner's A Time to Dance (1998), directed by Brownwell & Wilcoxen, produced by BTI Films

Pioneering dance/movement therapist, Norma Canner gives a glimpse into her life work and experiences in this well-crafted film. It can be watched on BTI Film's Vimeo channel: https://vimeo.com/206250642.

Dead Poets Society (1989), directed by Peter Weir and produced by Touchstone Pictures

Dead Poets Society reminds us of the power of written, spoken and read work in bringing camaraderie, unspoken communication, and emotion to education, companionship, and internal freedom.

Good Will Hunting (1997), directed by Gus Van Sant and produced by Miramax Films.

Good Will Hunting reminds us that there are many ways of learning, we all have gifts to share, and we may choose to share those gifts in varying degrees.

The Color Purple (1985), directed by Steven Spielberg and produced by Warner Bros. Pictures.

The Color Purple shares a story of darkness and joy, literacy and illiteracy, and the power of human connection. In addition to the film, we also recommend the book, or the Broadway theater performance under the same name. In 2023, a musical version of the film, directed by Blitz Bazawule and produced again by Steven Spielberg and Quincy Jones along with the Broadway musical producers Scott Sanders and Oprah Winfrey, was released by Warner Bros. Pictures.

Organizations

International Federation of Poetry/Bibliotherapy: https://ifbpt.org/

The International Federation of Poetry/Bibliotherapy provides information about the field, training opportunities, and how to earn credentials as a poetry therapist.

References

Brownwell, I., & Wilcoxen, W. (Directors) (1998). *A time to dance: The life and work of Normal Canner* [Film; streaming]. BTI Films, Bushy Theater. https://vimeo.com/206250642

Carvalho, M., de Miranda, J., Gratier, M, da Silva, H. (2019). The impact of maternal voice in the fetus: A systematic review. *Current Women's Health Reviews, 15*(3), 196–206.

Demaine, K. (2022). *The roots and rhythm of the heart: Our musical connection to identity, sprit, and lineage*. Lightning Source.

Fish, B. (2019). Response art in art therapy: Historical and contemporary overview. *Art Therapy: The Journal of the American Art Therapy Association, 36*(3), 122–132.

Ford, L. (2015, October 20). Two-thirds of the world's illiterate adults are women, report finds. *The Guardian.* https://www.theguardian.com/global-development/2015/oct/20/two-thirds-of-worlds-illiterate-adults-are-women-report-finds

Franklin, M. (2010). Affect regulation, mirror neurons, and the third hand: Formulating mindful empathetic art interventions. *Art Therapy: The Journal of the American Art Therapy Association, 27*(4), 160–167.

Gendling, E.T. (1978). *Focusing.* Everest House.

Hirst, D.J. (2005). Form and function in the representation of speech prosody. *Speech Communication, 46*(3–4), 334–347.

International Federation for Biblio/Poetry Therapy (2023). *Overview of training.* https://ifbpt.org/overview-of-training/

Knill, P., Barba, H, & Fuchs, M. (1995). *Minstrels of the soul: Intermodal expressive therapy*. Palmerston Press.

Maslow, A. (1954). *Motivation and personality*. Harper and Brothers.

Nash, G. (2020). Response art in art therapy practice and research with a focus on reflecting peace imagery. *The International Journal of Art Therapy, 25*(1), 1–10.

Nin, A. (1981). *The diary of Anais Nin* (Vol. 7, 1966–1974). Mariner Books Classics.

Van Es, B. (2010). "Johannes fac Totum"?: Shakespeare's first contact with the acting companies. *Shakespeare Quarterly, 61*(4), 551–577.

White, E.B., & Williams, G. (1952). *Charlotte's web*. Harper & Brothers.

Woodward, S. (2019). Fetal, neonatal, and early infant experiences of maternal singing. In D. Howard, J. Nix, & G. Welch (Eds.), *The Oxford handbook of singing* (pp. 431–453). Oxford University Press.

Chapter 2

Cultivating Practice in Writing with Other Art Forms

Krystal Leah Demaine and Tamar Reva Einstein

Welcome Mat: This chapter will discuss the diverse ways in which different kinds of writing can be used in intermodal expressive arts therapy and will outline types of expressive writing. A broad discussion will be presented on the inclusion of expressive and creative writing processes in therapeutic work. Readers will be introduced to writing as improvisation and as non-judgmental free playing with words. Writing practice in its many forms will be addressed as well as where people write. Just as Goldberg (1990) refers to writing practice as a way of bringing us back to our unique selves.

Setting the Tone: The Blank Page, the Empty Stage

There are many diverse ways in which people warm up, focus, and make space for the writing experience. The places and locations where we write can play a role in our contemplation and stimulation of writing topics. For example, some people enjoy writing in public spaces like cafes, train stations, trains, the beach, a garden, parks, museums, aquariums, or at a bench on the curb of a busy city street. Some writers choose total isolation, like Thoreau who built a cabin in the woods to completely isolate himself from all humans to be surrounded by nature. In a 1982 interview with the British Broadcasting Company (BBC), children's author of *Charlie and the Chocolate Factory*, *Matilda*, and *James and the Giant Peach*, Roald Dahl shared with viewers his small writing shed which he built in the backyard of his England home (Ashmore, 2018). In this space, which he referred to as a hut, he was able to draw the window shades and keep out the sounds of the hustle and the bustle inside his family home.

Many of us write at home, in a space we designate for this sacred time. Our students and group participants are, by the nature of teaching environments, often asked to write in large groups, though they are focused on their own contained notebook or journal. The intimacy of writing is held and even inspired by being part of that writing community. We encourage sharing, and reading

DOI: 10.4324/9781003391876-3

parts aloud so that feedback and witnessing are an organic part of the tone of the space.

The Writers Critic and Writers Block

Many students, clients, and participants arrive with an art form that is their mother tongue or comfort zone. One of the things that is encouraged is for them to play with and explore outside their familiar art forms. This might be considered learning a new language that enables the soul to speak and express. For example, asking the poet to take a dance class or the musician to take a painting workshop. This expands one's ability to mix new colors on a palette, improvise new sounds with musical instruments and the voice, and combine found objects that until that moment had never met.

In expressive arts therapy training when we witness a person dance or move, we may consider how the environment—the stage set, the lighting, the music, or even silent pauses—may bring a sense of total expression. When people decide to train as expressive arts therapists, depending on in what part of the world they are studying, there are different requirements for their prior artistic training and abilities. As an artist, in any art form, there is a natural experience of practice and ritual in developing proficiency. On the other hand, many people have experienced the studies of art forms as competitive, judgmental, and technique-oriented. Nancy Scherlong (personal communication, November 15, 2023), a therapist and writer amongst many other things, shares that,

> When people in the healing arts think of writing as cranial, or like an intellectual add-on, it is like a rock in my shoe. Writing is no more from the head than music lives in the ears. The soul gets involved, the senses come alive, and time folds in on itself. It takes the whole universe to bring forward a story and sometimes years before it hits an audience or the page.

Our students have shared with us how traumatized they have felt by the judgmental tone of voice of certain training programs; programs in which the soul perhaps has been mislaid or forgotten. Part of what we do when we incorporate writing with other arts as a practice is unlearning the critical and judgmental aspect of how practice was offered or taught to our participants. As lovers of language and people who pay attention to words, we are hyper-focused on the meaning of words. We do not use the word critique when there is an exhibition, presentation, performance, or shared moment as we are focused on the process and practice not an expected outcome. Indeed, at the beginning of the year, we discuss the use of words with our students with the intent of being aware of the words that we choose. Etymonline (n.d.) defines the word critique as a "critical examination or review of the merits of something" which was restored from the

1702 French term critic defined as "art of criticism" and the Greek, *kritike* "the critical art." This resonates with how we are not looking for perfection and proficiency when we refer to writing *practice*. Akin to brushing your teeth and eating; writing and making art becomes a natural embodied part of one's life.

As a reminder, this book encourages free writing, "mistake" making, and creative expression; there are no mistakes in art, and there are no mistakes in writing. We can say, there is only right writing!

In Tamar's memory, during a class in the 1980s, one of her mentors compared *writer's block* with the word *fasting*. So, instead of looking at not being capable of writing, painting, dancing, or making music as being stuck in quicksand, perhaps one can reframe this terrible feeling of not doing it *write*, as your body, soul, and spirit need to *fast* from this art form. As we know, fasting is intermittent and occurs in many religions as a cleansing ritual. Maybe we do on occasion need to cleanse ourselves from an art form and then go back to it. One of the gifts of engaging in many art forms is that if I am fasting from one, I can move to a different one. This, by the way, allows the spirit to be nourished differently and is a wonderful topic to write about once you're freed from quicksand!

Taking the Fear Out of Writing

Some people are afraid to write. This leads us to invent gentle, playful, and sensitive writing invitations that slowly develop the acceptance and ownership of their writing. Because of our roots in expressive arts therapy, we use many art forms to warm up the groups before the writing begins. This can include body-oriented exercises like breathing, tapping, self-massage, visualization, stretching, trading seats, and walking around the room, just to name a few. In our classes and workshops, we then begin the writing. This can include writing single alphabetic letters repetitively on a page, then, after that, words; perhaps associative words, observational words, emotions, thoughts, and feelings; afterward, we might suggest writing intuitive and honest words, sentences, and phrases about their feelings about writing. For example: *I hate this exercise, This reminds me of grade school,* or *I cannot write,* the repetitive sentences sometimes are more optimistic: *I love this, I missed writing, I write every day.* Also, it is worth mentioning that some refuse to write at all, or immediately write a perfect poem, or admit to feeling that this is very foreign to them, but they are willing to take a step on this journey paved in letters. We hope that our students are then slowly freer to become part of the world of writing practice; indeed, we have found that to be true. We even, over oceans and countries, find that students thank us at the end of the year for inviting them to reread and summarize their course journals in academic and reflective papers. The initial fear of writing has transformed into a healthy and happy relationship with pen on paper. For students who have been disheartened and disillusioned by writing, it is our job to make it attractive again; to welcome them into the magical, transformative, and soulful world of writing.

Choosing Writing Materials: The Soothing Sounds of Pencils, Pens, and Typewriters

Writers are invited to use a pen, pencil, crayon, marker, typewriter, or computer, whatever they feel most comfortable with when writing. Our personal preference, what may be considered old fashioned, is using a notebook with pen or pencil; allowing writers to write, doodle in the margins, and even cross out words, as opposed to deleting them, so that they can see their process.

The sound of a pencil swishing across the paper, zzzzshhh, zzzzshhh, especially in the silence of a room with no speaking becomes a unique yet calming soundscape for us as facilitators to witness. The engaging act of penning eludes talking and simply employs the swishing and whirring of the manual pencil or pen. It also allows for people's penmanship and writing to emerge.

Tick, Tick, Bing! Remembering the Typewriter

For those of you who remember or who don't, writers used to write with typewriters. First, they were manual and then electric. When writing with a typewriter, like when writing by hand, you can see your so-called mistakes. With a typewriter, one had to white out a mistake which was either with a white liquid or a little white tab that was inserted into the typewriter that allowed the mistake to be erased and retyped over. The once familiar sound of the typewriter pales in comparison with the computer where there is typically much less audible sound, perhaps sometimes clanking, but the typewriter with its, tick, tick, tick, tick bing!, tick tick tick bing!, leaves an aural imprint!

It turns out that there are still people who love, collect, and use typewriters. For example, the famous actor Tom Hanks is obsessed with them. In an article published in *Far Out Magazine*, Hanks was reported to own 250 typewriters for which he noted pleasure in its sounds and the ease of their maintenance (Russell, 2022). Hanks loves the machine so much that he even worked with techies to create an app called *Hanx Writer* that can turn your phone or tablet instantly into a clickety-clackety-sounding typewriter!

Perhaps it is the generation of authors that we love, but we have found that the famous authors who use the typewriter find something special or magical in the sensory experience the machine arouses. According to the *Harvard Business Review*, novelist Danielle Steele has a passion for typewriters with which she has written more than 170 novels and children's stories (Beard, 2022). Similarly, according to *The New York Times*, author Cormac McCarthy used a manual typewriter to write all of his work from the 1960s to 2009 (Cohen, 2009).

Going back to the pen and pencil, and in *Writing Down the Bones*, Natalie Goldberg (1986) suggests:

> First, consider the pen you write with. It should be a fast-writing pen because your thoughts are always much faster than your hand. You don't want to slow up your hand even more with a slow pen. A ballpoint, a pencil, and a felt tip, for sure, are slow. Go to a stationery store and see what feels good to you. Try out different kinds. Don't get too fancy and expensive. I mostly use a cheap Sheaffer fountain pen, about $1.95... You want to be able to feel the connection and texture of the pen on paper.
>
> (p. 5)

In summary, one can experiment and write with many tools of the trade, from ballpoint pen, to spray paint, to pencils, typewriters, markers, stencils, stamps, embroidered letters, collage letters, and whatever other writing whim takes you on your journey.

Improvisation and Playing with Words

Growing up, we were taught not to play with our food. We probably did. Now we invite you to cover yourself, without a bib, in mushy letters, mashed words, and soupy sentences. Please, play with your words!

In much of the education system globally we have noticed that very young children are encouraged to write. It seems that the learning of letter writing and reading has been implemented progressively earlier. There is a rapid evolution of literacy in some parts of the world. According to the Literacy Project Foundation website (2019), most children in the United States learn to read around the age of seven but are introduced to letter writing around the age of three or four while in nursery school where the emphasis on the rules of reading and writing comes before the improvisational part of writing. These writing conventions occur at an age when children are still fully engaged in playing naturally and developmentally. In a way, children are being asked to draw within the lines and write without going into the margin.

Our observation about reading and writing rules and regulations coming before creative play and improvisation is based on teaching both undergraduate and graduate college students who find creative writing to be a brand-new language or one that they have not engaged with in such a long time that it has built up a metaphorical rust that needs removal.

As a personal example, when Krystal began studying music at the age of eight, she was taught strictly in baroque and classical styles which contained specific rules according to her instructor. She was trained to read music exactly the way it was composed on the sheet of music, and this grade school child expected that if she practiced enough when she returned to her private lesson a week later, she would know the musical piece perfectly as written. This example is being given from the world of music; however, many people have experienced similar art education in all of the arts, including writing, which is why it is so hard to allow flow and spontaneity in our adult lives when we create in the arts. It is important to mention that as Krystal developed and studied the music of other genres including jazz, Latin, and blues, she realized that there was a whole other way to learn and study music. The moral of this story is to not let your past arts education stop you from experimenting, expanding, and learning new ways to become re-enchanted with the arts.

Rituals of Writing: Journaling, Diary Keeping, Altered Books

When referring to rituals of writing some people may refer to the term as writing practice or daily practice. As author, Terry Tempest Williams said (1984), "Rituals are the formulas by which harmony is restored" (p. 169). In Buddhism, daily practice is used and is transferred to other non-Buddhist rituals that are done daily. In the art world, daily practice can also include any of the arts; we will be focusing on writing. As Ralph Waldo Emerson (1870) said, "Write it on your heart that every day is the best day in the year" (p. 157). In our understanding, the best day of the year doesn't have to be the brightest, sunniest, or most beautiful, it can be that we are grateful that we woke up, we are breathing, and we can write. Perhaps, we might say, *write from your heart*. Writing comes in many forms, shapes, and sizes. Some people keep dream journals for decades, and some people keep diaries that travel with them. Some folks don't write daily but write regularly as it suits their schedule and abilities. Fuchs Knill and Atkins (2020) wrote that "a daily practice of poetry writing often brings surprises and new learning" (p. 43). This is important to mention because daily writing doesn't work for everyone. Practice, in our terminology for this book, refers to writing and perhaps adding other art forms, in a regular and ongoing manner that does not add pressure to writing. Returning to Buddhism, the idea of daily practice is meant to be a calming ritual, not an anxiety-provoking one.

If you are one of those people who write daily or if you are one of those people who wishes they would write daily, or if you are somewhere in between, all of that is acceptable and very commendable! On a personal note, Tamar, since 2017, has painted a watercolor every morning when she wakes up. She reprimanded herself for not keeping a daily journal or having a daily practice for decades. When the time was right in the seasons of her life, her daily painting practice began organically. The daily paintings have taken directions that were not intended or planned, friends and family became curious, and slowly the images were sent out to two separate groups of people, some only on Friday, as requested, and at times written responses are received. Two friends have begun their daily writing practice as responses to the paintings, one friend gives the watercolor an imaginary name and the other friend writes a poem in response to the painting each day. Tamar still has the private wish to also write a poem a day but has not gotten there yet. She writes three poems weekly in the spiritual poetry writing class she belongs to; a community of writers who are connected deeply to one another and their spiritual poems. The poets are from different religious and spiritual backgrounds and diverse geographic places. Poetry is the connecting glue in these sacred weekly meetings. A ritual that Tamar waits for each week.

Journaling and Diary Keeping

Journaling and diary-keeping have been put together in this section because we see overlaps in these two writing formats. In both, some folks only write, or write and add visuals. Some people write in their journals and diaries daily, some weekly, some in cycles, and some leave for long durations of time and then go back to them. Some people strive to write in their journals daily.

People keep journals for many reasons: secret telling, documentation, affirmation, reminders of gratitude, working through traumas, dream journals, during rites of passage, for remembering ideas, anthropological notes, ancestral stories, research journals, and most simply for self-reflection. When things are broken, we write. When there is an obstacle, it makes us want to write. Like in a book, the pages of the writing of our life stories are glued and threaded together at the spine; that magical place that keeps us up*write* no matter what we are going through.

Though Tamar does not keep a daily diary (she has tried but it somehow never sticks), she does deeply love reading other people's published diaries and journals. This began early on. She was gifted, by a beloved cousin, the diaries of Anaïs Nin (1966–1977) at age 12, which might seem young for such erotic literature; she was simultaneously reading *Harriet the Spy* (Fitzhugh, 1964), whose heroine famously kept a diary. This combination was perfect for Tamar at that age, for her. All of the books have been reread over and over at different times in her life; each time harvesting new fruits and wisdom. Both Anaïs Nin and Harriet, like Mary Poppins and Pippi Longstocking, are female role models that Tamar keeps on her bookshelves today. They are sandwiched between Collette, *Charlotte's Web*, and Isabella Allende's books. They never grow old, just dog-eared and better.

One of the most widely sold diaries printed in 52 languages and read by millions worldwide is Anne Frank's diary which was written while she was hiding from the Nazis during World War II (Frank, 1952/1989). One can imagine that this kind of diary-keeping is almost a survival technique and a way of leaving documentation behind after war atrocities occur and people are murdered. Frank was not a historian, she was not a politician, she was a real person who wrote about real things and this may be why her diary has touched so many people across the world. Diaries are a safe container for the deepest feelings from optimism and pessimism, to fear and hope. On July 15, 1944, Anne Frank (1952/1989) wrote in her journal:

> I see the world being slowly transformed into a wilderness, I hear the approaching thunder that, one day, will destroy us too, and I feel the suffering of millions. And yet, when I look up at the sky, I somehow feel that everything will change for the better that this cruelty too shall end, that peace and tranquility will return once more.
>
> (pp. 276–277)

John Steinbeck talks about the fact that if you want to write as a practice you have to get up and do it. In Steinbeck's (1990) *Working Days, Journals of The Grapes of Wrath,* there is no saying, *I am not getting up today to write*:

> In writing, habit seems to be a much stronger force than either willpower or inspiration. Consequently, there must be some little quality of fierceness until the habit pattern of a certain number of words is established. There is no possibility, in me at least, of saying, "I'll do it if I feel like it." One never feels like working day after day. In fact, given the smallest excuse, one will not work at all. The rest is nonsense. Perhaps some people can work that way, but I cannot. I must get my words down every day whether they are any good or not.
>
> (p. 119)

As Natalie Goldberg (1986) reminds us in her rules of writing practice. Rule number six says:

> You are free to write the worst junk in *America*, you can be more specific if you like; the worst junk in Santa Fe; New York; Kalamazoo, Michigan; your city block; your pasture; your neighborhood restaurant; your family. Or you can get more cosmic: free to write the worst junk in the universe, galaxy, world, hemisphere, Saraha Desert.
>
> (p. 4)

Inspired by Natalie Goldberg, we remind our students to do it [write] every day even if your writing is terrible; it is the practice that counts. In her current online writing workshops, Goldberg (2023) continues to reiterate the sentiment to just write; without judgment and without allowing what she refers to, in Buddhism, as the *monkey mind*, to get in the way of your writing process. Most importantly, writing is a practice and we need to write regularly, no matter what comes out.

In his diary, Franz Kafka (1990/2022) talks about looking back at our journals and realizing our difficulties and how we get through them; Kafka realized strengths in ourselves through reflection:

> In the diary, you find proof that in situations that today would seem unbearable, you lived, looked around, and wrote down observations, that this right hand moved then as it does today, when we may be wiser because we can look back upon our former condition, and for that very reason have got to admit the courage of our earlier striving in which we persisted even in sheer ignorance.
>
> (p. 145)

The journaling and diary writing examples that we have chosen to focus on in this section are comparatively quite different in their content, yet, similar in their writing habit continuity. In other words, when people keep diaries and journals it is or becomes inseparable from their daily soul nourishment. It is a meal that one cannot miss.

Dream Journaling

In many forms of therapy, it is considered important to keep dream journals. In other words, to write down one's dreams, or, in this day and age, as Tamar does, to record them into your phone when you wake up from your dream. These dreams are then analyzed, interpreted, and looked at closely for symbols and themes, depending on the dream analysis theory that the therapist has been trained in. For example, Carl Jung (1929) said, "In sleep, fantasy takes the form of dreams. But in waking life, too, we continue to dream beneath the threshold of the consciousness" (p. 125). Some therapists ask their clients to draw their dreams, but what we are talking about here is written dream journals.

Dreams, as some infer, can among other things be hidden wishes or hopes for the future, just as the Everly Brothers sang, in their song titled, *All I Have to Do is Dream* (Bryant, 1958). According to Benetez-Eves (2021), songwriters for decades have used inspiration from their dreams to write many of their lyrics. Sometimes these dreams are written about daydreams, or sometimes during what Jungians refer to as lucid dreams; dreaming is not limited to a deep night's rest on the pillow, as noted by The Monkees, in their song, *Daydream Believer* (Stewart, 1967).

According to an article penned in *Autobiography Magazine*, the brilliant musician and songwriter, Paul McCartney, gave an interview in 1988 describing how he composed the well-known song *Yesterday* in his sleep (Zakarin, 2020). When he woke up, he went straight over to the piano transcribed the melody, and then added lyrics to the well-known song.

On a different dreamscape and a non-musical note, author Mary Shelley (1818/1984) wrote the book *Frankenstein* based on a nightmare she had about building a creature from dismembered corpses. The dream haunted her so much that she woke up frantically and began writing down her story (Marriott, 2017).

Barbara Black Koltuv (2011), clinical psychologist and Jungian analyst, wrote about dreamwork,

> Simply writing down dreams, and allowing them to matter, opens a way. Human beings need meaning, just as we need food, *water,* and *air*. Without it, we suffer dreadful loneliness, alienation, depression, and anxiety. When we begin to pay attention to dreams, a symbol system, a personal mythology, and soul language comes into being.
>
> (p. 3)

While Freud commonly discussed his work with his clients in his books, he also wrote about his dreams in his seminal book *The Interpretation of Dreams* (1900/2010). His way of working with dreams was by specific symbolic interpretation and analysis. In Freud's (1908/1995) "Creative Writers and Day-Dreaming," he said of creative writers and daydreaming, "A piece of creative writing, like a daydream, is a continuation of, and a substitute for, what was once the play of childhood" (p. 19).

According to the Museum of Modern Art's website (n.d.) on the topic of surrealism and the subconscious,

> Freud and other psychoanalysts used a variety of techniques to bring to the surface the subconscious thoughts of their patients. The Surrealists borrowed many of the same techniques to stimulate their writing and art, with the belief that the creativity that came from deep within a person's subconscious could be more powerful and authentic than any product of conscious thought.
>
> (para 1)

Liza Hyatt, a licensed art therapist and natural dreamwork practitioner who works with people in a different way than Jungian or Freudian practitioners, shared:

> Here is the writing process I use to do my own dreamwork. It is the same process I encourage my dreamwork clients to cultivate... To engage in Natural Dreamwork, I write my dreams into a digital dream journal... I write my dream narratives in the present tense so that they feel as if they are still active and alive. I focus on describing in vivid detail the images, feelings, and interactions in the dream—what I sensed, felt, said, and who I met in the dream... Putting in as much specific detail helps me more vividly

remember the dream and be able to embody it in my dreamwork sessions. It respects the dream as a rich and mysterious experience. I do not explain the dream or add assumptions.... My dream worker will give me moments from the dream to focus on as meditative homework between sessions. We will write these dream moments down and I will add them to my digital dream journal... This way of maintaining my journal helps me trace the path of the profound soul work and healing that engaging in dreamwork as a spiritual practice offers.

(personal communication, December 1, 2023)

Altered Books

If you are old enough, you might remember getting your clothing altered at a tailor. We define the word alter as changed. When discussing altered books, we use the word alter to mean many ways of changing or transforming a book in a significant way. This change can occur in many small ways, in destruction and reconstruction, with additions and subtractions, burning, sewing, gluing, drawing, painting, buttoning, cutting, piercing, folding, adding writing, removing writing, blackout poetry, using gesso, blanking out pages, using only the cover or using only the pages inside, adding envelopes, pockets, drawers, or secret doors. Adding found objects like locks, buttons, clocks, or other objects that protrude from the book. These are just some of the many possible examples of how one can alter a book.

Altered books are, as far as we are concerned, an extremely accessible creative way to connect to writing alongside and with many other art forms in a contained space, a book. One personal example Tamar can share is of an altered book that was part of an unforgettable, sacred artmaking time with a dear friend who was dying. This experience was shared with another friend, who is an artist and spiritual caregiver, the three were very close. It began with the dear friend saying she, at times, wished she could create a cocoon, in one of our weekly visits to her home. This turned into us playing with art supplies together and alone as we sat around a round wooden table, making container-like objects. As she withered away each week, the notion of a shared-altered book arose over tea. The other friend and Tamar went looking for books at a public space where folks leave books out for the taking. They simultaneously found four copies of the same book on two separate sides of this space. When they met in the middle, they looked at each other and knew, THIS WAS THE BOOK. Kismet? Synchronicity? Beshert? Spiritual connection? Call it what you'd like, but they believed it was no accident. For a couple of months, they each worked on their copies, but there was one that went between them, round robin, in which each week one took the book and added to it. Sometimes responding to the others, sometimes not. They pasted, embroidered, tore, cut, wrote, added, took away, and did everything and anything they felt was meaningful and right at that moment. Their beloved sick friend worked with them creating art weekly, including in the book, until the Sunday of the week she died. They were asked to bring the book to the funeral and say a few words about how alive she became when they were creating together. Her family now has that book. The last thing she added was a recipe card she found from her grandmother.

Altered books can be used by many professions for diverse reasons including research as Chilton (2013) stated, "I present altered book making and poetry as a process of imaginative inquiry into arts-based research" (p. 457). Using altered books as a form of arts-based research is familiar and heartwarming to Tamar who created an altered research book as she moved forward throughout the doctoral process. Altered books also offer deep introspective reframing of life stories and narratives, grief work, and identity work, for example. These books are not as new as one might expect, according to Cobb and Negash (2010), altered books have a history going far back in time:

> The history of altering books can be traced back to the 11th century when the scarcity of paper encouraged Italian monks to recycle old vellum manuscripts. By scraping the ink off of old books and recovering the pages with new text and illustrations, new books were created.
>
> (p. 59)

This is a wonderful example of how creativity comes alive when problem-solving arises. In our minds, this image of the monks scraping ink meticulously is inspiring and such a great discovery to share with our students when they are trained on how to use altered books in expressive therapies, both for themselves and their clients.

In the academic setting, Krystal uses altered books as a way for students to document their process throughout the 15-week-long semester. Students are instructed at the beginning of the semester to find a hardcovered book with many pages and lots of words. As a transformative art diary, students are invited into the book as a place to transform from the inside and outside, to alter text, cut, rip, tear, glue, tape, staple, draw, paint, and draw in whatever way transforms the words and meaning of the text. Some students choose to use their altered book to draw in the margins during class periods, to take notes, or to integrate non-traditional materials like makeup, perfumes, oils, nail polish, or tea, transforming the look, feel, and scent of the pages. Some students rewrite the table of contents and create new titles. Some students work on their books once a day and others do not. By the end of the semester the book has become their own, a place where their words are written; the text is cut and replaced, taken away, or folded over. A safe space encased between a spine and cover that has been redesigned. A book is a symbolic and literal process and product of owning one's narrative; a container with two sides hugging one's life story.

In another academic setting, set in the woods in Indiana, in a graduate art therapy program, Tamar and her friend and colleague Dr. Jill McNutt, who was the program director at the time, found themselves walking up a flight of beautiful antique wooden stairs to rooms on a floor once used as dormitories decades before. Pushing open a large wooden, brass-knobbed door of a room, they were astonished to be in the presence of piles and piles of ancient, dusty books. They looked at each other and immediately began rummaging through these long-forgotten treasures. They chose books for a class Tamar was teaching on studio arts and a couple for themselves. The books were schlepped downstairs, dusted off, and kept safely in Jill's office. Chilton (2007) wrote that, "Dusty old books may represent neglected or forgotten knowledge, or an earlier chapter of one's life. Opening or closing a book may symbolize opening or closing a stage in one's life" (p. 60).

When Tamar brought a pile of these books to the students on the first day of class and described how they could be altered, changed, and transformed, as the beginning of the process of the four-day face-to-face studio art class which would then be continued throughout the semester online, the participants' eyes lit up. They took time to choose books, some were chosen because of illustrations, some because they were crumbling, some because their spines were broken, and some because there were titles that appealed to them. The first assignment was to re-create the cover. This began a creative process that Tamar found astonishing, truly enchanting. One woman covered the cover with clay and daily watched the cracking and changing, one collaged, one used nature objects, one painted, and one highlighted the title that was already embossed in gold on the cover. Then, the work on the interiors began: tearing, gluing, blacking out poetry, painting, adding pockets, embroidering, cutting big spaces out to create inner containing spaces, and folding techniques, which are just some examples of what was done.

The discussions during and at the closing of each day were full of self-discoveries, playful banter, serious tragic narratives, and deep sharing. All aspects of life seem to be contained and held in these books as they were created. The books reappeared at different points online in the course discussion boards, the writing about them was moving, freeing, cathartic, and surprising, according to the students. The penning of words brought clarity, focus, and affirmation to the process and product. An unforgettable altered book academic experience for all. Tamar felt the retelling and transformation through the writing; she too was transformed by these incredible students.

Altered books, it must be mentioned, are not easily digested by all clients and students. Many people have a strong aversion to what they call "destroying" a book. Depending on one's cultural, economic, geographic, and religious upbringing, books can carry a sacred meaning. This is very understandable, and one is not to be pushed beyond places that are not comfortable in therapy or classes. We can find other ways to get to similar outcomes, perhaps using magazines or welcoming the person to write about the feelings that have arisen; not taking for granted that all folks will find altering books a good match for them. We have noticed, throughout the years, that not one of our students, anywhere in the world, has ever chosen a holy religious book to alter. This is an important discussion to open with students and participants. Even artistic and poetic license have their boundaries.

Therapeutic Journaling

There is a professional field of journal therapy. One can become trained as a certified journal therapist. The Center for Journal Therapy website (2023) offers information and resources about the professional field of therapeutic journals, including links to their training division, the Therapeutic Writing Institute. Neither of us have done this training. We have been taught and trained through the expressive arts therapy education we received, to use writing, including journaling, in our work, clinically and academically.

Since the advent of social media and the internet, one might reach millions of people with the press of a button, literally, and sometimes by accident. One thing that we have observed is that people are sharing very personal things that they have written in very public spaces. This sharing seems to be the opposite of what diary keeping and journaling were when one was first acquainted with it. We have memories of journals that were given to us by family or friends that had beautiful covers and a tiny silver lock and key, to ensure privacy. Privacy and a safe space to write! Remember privacy, everyone? No password was needed, just a tiny key, that you also hid under your pillow, maybe in your underwear drawer, or in the bottom of your school bag.

What we mean to say is, that we try to instill the sanctity of personal and private writing in our work. We encourage journaling and diary keeping of any sort as a practice or not. Go ahead, write once a week, once a day, once a year, and take ownership of calling that your form of journaling or diary keeping. We also believe in self-care and taking pauses, just as Maya Angelou (Martell, 2010) described in her practice of taking Saturday for herself.

Writing Invitations

1 **Haiku: Mother Nature Reflection**
   Haikus are short poems with a general focus on nature. They do not need to rhyme. You may use the traditional 5–7-5 meter to write your haiku or you can choose to write (in honor of Natalie Goldberg) just *Three Simple Lines* (Goldberg, 2021). We suggest first choosing an object from nature: a leaf, a stone, a body of water, a feather, or a bone. Hold the object in your hand and mentally note its texture, shape, form, color, and weight. Write your haiku in reflection of this nature element, and other nature elements just as you experience them. We invite you to find some haiku to read and become inspired.

2   Aesthetic Response to Haiku

The British Museum published a book called *Haiku Animals* (Pilbeam, 2010) in which every few pages illustrates a beautiful Japanese painting of an animal alongside a haiku written about that animal in both Japanese and English transliteration. We are amazed how haiku can illustrate a whole word in three lines. We invite you to think of two animals, either those that you are very familiar with or know nothing about, and write a three-line haiku about them. Here are two haikus that we think are brilliant. One haiku is written by the classic haiku writer Shiki and the other is written by Buson.

1   Writing Sounds

In Chapter 2, we discussed the *tick, tick, bing!* sound of the typewriter and the *zzzzshhh* of the pencil swishing across the paper as our students wrote on their papers in a quiet group. Think of a sound that crosses your daily path when all other things are quiet; perhaps windshield wipers oscillating, the humming of a refrigerator, the flickering buzz of an incandescent lamp. Write about the sound quality, its frequency, pitch, tonality, vibrato, and perhaps its crescendo or cadence. Perhaps you move the sound into the musical sphere as you explore writing sounds.

2   Blackout Poetry

In altered bookmaking, one might decide to focus on blackout poetry. Our way of doing this is as follows. Choose a book that you can work in, knowing that it will be forever changed like indelible ink changes a surface. The search for the book is sometimes as meaningful as the finding of the right book. Once found, begin looking at a page, you can choose randomly and or go in chronological order. Use all pages of the book. Maybe a date on the first page calls out to you, or a handwritten inscription. Seek out words that speak to you, that want attention, that resonate with how you feel at that moment. Make a thin pencil line around those words to delineate them before the blacking out begins. There can be few or many words chosen. Then take a black marker, (place a piece of cardboard or baking paper underneath so the black ink doesn't seep through to the next pages, unless that feels right to you in your process), and black out the unneeded words, and leave the ones you circled with pencil. You will end up with a black page with your chosen words standing out. Do this throughout the entire book. Afterward, reread the words, see if themes emerged, decorate and ornament the front and back covers in response to the themes, and title your new book, that you, and only you, have created.

3   Dream Words

Using a dream you have had, old or new, night dreamed or daydreamed, create a list of words that are associated with the dream. Descriptive words, nouns, prepositions, verbs, adjectives, and adverbs. Then after creating this list, write each word on a card, maybe an index card or cards you prepare from heavy paper. On the other side of the card, find an image from a magazine or online and glue it on, or draw your illustration. Once finished keep them in a box, which you can ornament as well, in any way you choose. Take the cards out and move them around, placing them in different ways, like a mosaic of words. What appears? Look and write on a separate page in a notebook using the connected words as raw material for a new narrative, a new story... You may add as many words as needed for this to come together and make sense. Try the same process with the images and write about them. Your dream is the foundation for creating and reframing a new tale.

Resources

Places

Walden Pond State Reservation, 915 Walden Street, Concord, MA, USA

Meander, explore, swim, hike, or fish, the more than 460 acres of Walden Pond State Reservation where Henry David Thoreau's book, *Walden* was inspired. You can also visit a replica of Thoreau's writing cabin while on the grounds.

Articles

In an interview by Noelle Oxenhandler, published online in *Lion's Roar* on September 28, titled "The Zen of Jane Hirschfield," Hirschfield compares and describes her writing practice and her meditation practice. She discusses deep listening and accepting liminal space. You an access it here: https://www.lionsroar.com/zen-jane-hirshfield/.

Websites

The Natural Dreamwork website introduces a phenomenological approach to working with dreams, with a guide, which helps one to have a more intimate relationship with images that arise in dreams. This includes writing. You can access it here: https://www.thenaturaldream.com/.

Videos

If you want to make your own altered books, the following YouTube videos show steps and ideas on how to make and create them. These diverse tutorials open doors to the many ways one can alter a book with both different kinds of writing and the arts.

- Spirit of Nature Art (2022, September 30). *Find your own rhythm – altered book art journal tutorial* [Video]. YouTube. https://www.youtube.com/watch?v=0ddXqZeKa7o

- Creative Soul Journeys (2022, January 12). *Altered book art journal: Make something old new again* [Video]. YouTube. https://www.youtube.com/watch?v=QHkr7PWrT2Y
- Lein-Svencner, L. (2022, November 30). *Altered books and altered writing journals* [Video]. YouTube. https://www.youtube.com/watch?v=T_E1e2whjHI
- Mr Spencer ELA (2020, April 25). *Blackout poetry: A completed lesson* [Video]. YouTube. https://www.youtube.com/watch?v=Ub6KDCIt_cY

Sound researcher Julian Treasure offers five suggestions that may be useful for exploring sound in his July 2011 TED talk, 5 Ways to Listen Better. Here is a link to it: https://www.ted.com/talks/julian_treasure_5_ways_to_listen_better?language=en.

Natalie Goldberg offers her thoughts on writing haiku in an interview by Tara Brach, titled, "Tara Brach interviews Natalie Goldberg: Writing and haiku as spiritual practice." It can be seen on Brach's YouTube channel, uploaded on July 28, 2021: https://www.youtube.com/watch?v=o7BLrezIfHA&t=1s

Natalie Goldberg also shares her thoughts on Dharma Talk in this 2023 Upaya Zen Center video found on their YouTube channel. It is titled: "Zazen and Dharma Talk with Natalie Goldberg: Haiku – the leap" and was published on March 22: https://www.youtube.com/watch?v=PInw2EV1wsE.

In this 2021 interview from the Mountain Cloud Zen Center, Natalie Goldberg shares her three simple lines exercise. Titled "An evening with Natalie Goldberg: Three simple lines" and shared on January 14, 2021, on their YouTube channel, it can be viewed at: https://www.youtube.com/watch?v=zWNBtokzobg.

Applications

Inspired by world-famous actor, Tom Hanks, the Hanx Writer is an application designed to give your cell phone or tablet keys the sounds of a typewriter! You can learn more about it on their website: http://hanxwriter.com/. To see a demonstration of it, check out this video, "Tom Hanks' Hanx Writer App Demo," uploaded on August 18, 2014, to the TechCrunch YouTube channel: https://www.youtube.com/watch?v=Z3dvZSSqCj8.

References

Ashmore, C. [Telling Tales with Carl Ashmore]. (2018, January 31). *Roald Dahl interview and short film – Pebble Mill at One 1982* [Video]. YouTube. https://www.youtube.com/watch?v=nQkz_X1Rg60

Beard, A. (2021). Life's work: An interview with Danielle Steele. *Harvard Business Review*. https://hbr.org/2021/11/lifes-work-an-interview-with-danielle-steel

Benetez-Eves, T. (2021). *15 Songs that were written from dreams*. American Songwriter: The Craft of Music. https://americansongwriter.com/15-songs-that-were-written-from-dreams/

Black Koltuv, B. (2011). *Nights at the wall: A guide to dreams, dreamwork, and profound self-knowledge.* Nicolas Hays Incorporated.

Bryant, B. (1958). *All I have to do is dream [Song recorded by the Everly Brothers].* Acuff-Rose Music; RCA Studios Nashville.

Center for Journal Therapy. (2023). *Do you want to journal?* https://journaltherapy.com/

Chilton, G. (2007). Altered books in art therapy with adolescents. *Art Therapy, 24*(2), 59–63.

Chilton, G. (2013). Altered inquiry: Discovering arts-based research through an altered book. *International Journal of Qualitative Methods, 12*(1), 457–477.

Cobb, R.A., & Negash, S. (2010). Altered bookmaking as a form of art therapy: A narrative approach. *Journal of Family Psychotherapy, 21*(1), 54–69.

Cohen, P. (2009, November 30). No country for old typewriters: A well-used one-heads to auction. *The New York Times.* https://web.archive.org/web/20200616052132/https://www.nytimes.com/2009/12/01/books/01typewriter.html

Emerson, R.W. (1870). *Society and solitude.* Fields, Osgood.

Etymonline. (n.d.). Critique (n.). In *Online etymology dictionary.* Retrieved December 15, 2023, from https://www.etymonline.com/search?q=critique

Fitzhugh, L. (1964). *Harriet the spy.* Harper & Row.

Freud, S. (1900/2010). *The interpretation of dreams.* Basic Books.

Freud, S. (1908/1995). Creative writers and day-dreaming. In P. Gay (Ed.), *The Freud reader* (Reissue ed., pp. 436–443). W. W. Norton & Company.

Goldberg, N. (1986). *Writing down the bones: Freeing the writer within.* Shambhala Publications.

Goldberg, N. (1990). *Wild mind: Living the writer's life.* Bantam Books.

Goldberg, N. (2021). *Three simple lines: A writer's pilgrimage into the heart and homeland of haiku.* New World Library.

Goldberg, N. (2023). Winter practice period: Dharma talk with Natalie Goldberg. *Upaya Meditation Center.* https://www.upaya.org/video/winter-practice-period-dharma-talk-with-natalie-goldberg-2023/

Jung, C.G. (1929). The problems of modern psychotherapy. In E.A. Read (Ed.), *The collected works of C. G. Jung* (Vol. 16). Princeton University Press.

Kafka, F. (1990/2022). *The Diaries of Franz Kafka, 1910–1923*, R. Benjamin (Trans.). Schocken.

Knill, M.F., & Atkins, S. (2020). *Poetry and expressive arts: Supporting resilience through poetry writing.* Jessica Kingsley Publishers.

Literacy Project Foundation (2019, February 14). 30 Key child literacy stats parents need to be aware of. *Literacy Project.* https://literacyproj.org/2019/02/14/30-key-child-literacy-stats-parents-need-to-be-aware-of/

Frank, A. (1952/1989). *The diary of Anne Frank.* Doubleday.

Marriott, L. (2017). Waking dreams and cadavers: Mary Shelly's *Frankenstein. Headstuff.* https://headstuff.org/culture/history/waking-dreams-mary-shelley-frankenstein/

Martell, N. (2010, November 10). Maya Angelou: An interview. *Washington City Paper.* https://washingtoncitypaper.com/article/429700/dr-maya-angelou-exclusive-interview/

Museum of Modern Art. (n.d.). Tapping the subconscious: Automatism and dreams. https://www.moma.org/collection/terms/surrealism/tapping-the-subconscious-automatism-and-dreams

Nin, Anaïs (1966–1977). *The diary of Anais Nin* (Vol. 1–7). Harcourt Brace Jovanovich.
Pilbeam, M. (2010). *Haiku animals.* British Museum Press.
Russell, C. (2022, May 3). Tom Hanks' wholesome obsession with typewriters. *Far Out Magazine.* https://faroutmagazine.co.uk/tom-hanks-obsession-typewriters/
Shelley, Mary (1818/1994). *Frankenstein* (3rd ed.). Dover Publications.
Steinbeck, J. (1990). *Working days: The journals of the grapes of wrath.* Penguin Books.
Stewart, J. (1967). *Daydream believer [Song recorded by the Monkees].* RCA Victor Studios; Colgems.
Williams, T.T. (1984). *Pieces of white shell: A journey to Navajoland.* UNM Press.
Zakarin, J. (2020, September 8). *Paul McCartney came up with the melody to one of the Beatles' biggest hits in his sleep.* Biography. https://www.biography.com/musicians/paul-mccartney-the-beatles-yesterday-dream

Chapter 3

Writing as Praising Common Things

Odes, Prayers, Hymns, Amulets, and Rituals

Krystal Leah Demaine and Tamar Reva Einstein

Welcome Mat: Honoring Pablo Neruda's "Ode to Common Things" (1994), this chapter expands the reader's creative writing palate and gets the juices flowing through the exploration of seemingly mundane objects as a springboard for writing. Readers and writers will build the link between visual representation to expressive writing. No prior art experience is necessary; come as you are, this pertains to all of the explorations in this book.

Setting the Space through Ritual

In expressive arts therapy, we are very aware that the place in which learning occurs needs to be differentiated from the outside world; we do this by using objects that signal to the participants or students that they have entered the sacred space of arts and healing. As essayist, historian, and philosopher, Tomas Carlyle (1838) wrote "In every object, there is inexhaustible meaning" (p. 5). This is the atmosphere in which odes, prayers, hymns, and amulets are written and created in our classes, groups, and workshops.

Before Krystal begins her groups, in the middle of the circle, while students or participants sit silently and watch her, she lays a large rectangular tapestry that has a colorful mandala printed on it. Krystal places the objects she has chosen that day slowly and meticulously on the fabric, which may include art materials, colorful organza scarves, musical instruments, flowers, singing bowls, rocks and stones, sea shells, postcards with images, scented materials, and sometimes food.

Cultivating a sanctity of safe space is a ritual that we have taken from our own studies and continue giving to our students, groups, and therapy clients. These traditions signal a rite of passage; the beginning of something, meaningful moments, or conclusions. In an example at The Phototherapy Institute in Jerusalem, Tamar and her very close friend and colleague created a closing ritual after the students shared their end-of-the-year photographs and processes. A long metal antique miniature bathtub was set up with flower petals floating on water. Each student was called up, handed a floating candle, asked to light it,

DOI: 10.4324/9781003391876-4

then to make a wish for the rest of their journey once the studies had ended, and finally place the candle to float in the water. Each student did this as the others and their families silently witnessed and listened intently. This was based on both Tamar and her colleague's studies in the 1980s at Lesley College where many of their classes began with the lighting of a large candle in the middle of the room, which Krystal and Tamar are no longer allowed to use in academic settings due to fire regulations about open flames. We lament the loss of candle lighting. That said, the light from the candles still shines within us and we pass it on to our students transformed into new rituals that work today, which sometimes utilize battery-operated flickering candles or a photograph of a candle. Nevertheless, the sacred space will always remain.

Writing About Common Things

Honoring Pablo Neruda's "Ode to Common Things" (1994), we help our students and participants get the writing juices flowing with sketching and drawing as a springboard for prose and poetry from the common objects in their daily lives. We are surrounded by objects every moment of the day from the moment we awaken to the moment we go to sleep. These objects might seem mundane or non-important, yet some might carry meaningful messages and stories. In our writing classes and workshops, we often invite people to express themselves about these objects through writing odes, psalms, prayers, and hymns to and about these objects alongside creations in other art forms.

After reading Neruda's poem "An Ode to Common Things" (1994), we ask our participants to do the following exercises. In a way, this is like writing an ode to Neruda's ode. An ode is almost a thank-you note. When we read Neruda's "Ode to Common Things" to our students, they are riveted.

Krystal has her students remove an object from their bag, something random, a thing that might always be there but is not noticed perhaps. Or one they are intimately familiar with, or one they may have forgotten or abandoned. They are then invited to draw a quick, associative, free-flow sketch, of this object. They can then write some thoughts, feelings, or descriptive observations down about the entire process. What new or surprising stories have emerged? Do they have a new connection to this object? A discussion closes the process.

In Tamar's version of this arts-based learning experience, phototherapy students are asked to bring objects that are related to photography from home and lay them out carefully on a shared table. They are then given 20 minutes to sketch from whatever angle of the table they choose, including sitting on the floor close to the edge of the table or far away. Photographers are often immersed in angles and light when they photograph. The physicality of sitting on the floor and looking up at a table gives the student a way to redirect these conversations between light and shadow: *chiaroscuro*, into drawing. The sketches are discussed, and the intermodal transfer is focused upon. Each student tells the origin story of the object that they brought to the class, as it relates to the reflective writing. What discoveries or connections have been made both to the student's object and the communal objects of others? How has the relationship between shadow and light, negative and positive space, affected the student's emotions as one moves from looking at the object to drawing the object?

We both use very similar techniques in different styles. Same language, different accent.

Odes

The origin of odes differs between historians and anthropologists. One of the theories is that odes originated in ancient Greece and were accompanied by music to celebrate athletes and their athletic victories. According to Tynianov and Shukman (2003), the word ode in English comes from the Greek *aeidein* meaning to chant or sing. Yet, odes exist in other ancient religious and belief systems. When we use odes in our teaching of writing, we look at them as a moment to pause, be mindful, carefully observe an object, and think about thanking this object for its existence. To take a moment to appreciate the object. We offer consideration for asking, what does this object give me? Why have I not paid attention to it in a deeper way? The writing allows the writer to form a deeper relationship with this often inanimate object.

Our students ask: *how does Neruda get from describing these common things and bringing them to a deeper personal connection, how do these objects play a role in his life, and how they have stirred him?* We then ask our students to write about an object; believing that writing about it will answer their own question.

In diverse spiritual and religious beliefs and practices being thankful for what we consider to be normal daily parts of our lives is practiced by blessings, sentences, chants, silent pauses, and meditations, which all relate to the act of gratitude. This includes blessings before and after eating food or drinking water, washing hands and other body parts, and after using the toilet, grateful that the body is working properly. There is also the practice of blessing beautiful scents; some thank yous are spoken out loud and some in silence. The reason we ask our students to engage in ode writing is we think that in therapy training it is extremely important to direct people to understand that there are many things we do not notice regularly. A therapist can be a person who reminds one, through their writing and arts-based work, to notice and be grateful for the minute details in their lives.

In other words, ode writing trains our students to pay attention to the details. Therapists need to hone their capabilities in focusing on details, such as a change in tone of voice, physical posture, and mannerisms in an objective and non-judgmental way. Honing in through writing invites our students also to learn to be grateful for the details. We hope that our students can use this practice in other ways as they move along their life journey; for self-reflection. In

Neurda's "Ode to Common Things," you can tell that his observational skills were exceptional. We hope that our observational skills and our students may be enhanced by such powerful poetry. Through the lens of photographer Wynn Bullock (1993), one can focus on creativity as an ode to life.

Prayers

When we use the word prayers in writing experientials, they are about asking for something, almost like making a wish. Often people come to therapy and sometimes to therapy training because they are going through extremely challenging times in their lives. Using writing, one can make up and create personal prayers, that can serve as anchors in the stormy times of life and that can tether the therapeutic experience. When one is invited to share aloud what prayers and wishes one needs and wants at the moment, there is a powerful moment of asking for help. In our experience, one of the hardest things for people to do is ask for help; especially out loud.

In our classes and in therapy, we create writing experiences that invite students, participants, and clients to write down these prayers and wishes, therefore documenting them and allowing them to be witnessed and affirmed. This process in itself can feel both freeing and anchoring. For the work we do, prayer is not connected to religiosity, though some people may find a connection to their spirituality or reconnection to new ways of thinking about what prayer might be in their lives. We believe that this kind of prayer writing, writing from the soul and the spirit, is as holy and sacred as any other prayer writing.

In our personal and professional experiences, as well as based on feedback from group participants (and not only those who are religious), when people are in deep darkness or grief they begin praying, asking for help, or making wishes. In these times, people look for an answer from another place they might have previously eschewed. Oftentimes, when people are going through a hard time they start praying; we ourselves have personally experienced this.

We have both experienced looking for a higher being, whatever word or term one might choose for that while sitting next to the beds of dying parents (Krystal's father and Tamar's mother, thousands of miles apart and in different years). This is another common thread that binds us together as we co-write this book. Similar incantations were murmured, whispered, cried, whimpered, sung silently, repeated, and said aloud by both of us with the wish that our parents' last journeys would be smooth and free of pain. As poet and priest John O'Donohue (2000) referred, in hard times prayer can offer a connection to those we have lost.

Hymns

We consider hymns to be poetry set to music. They are often poetic songs, sung aloud. Oftentimes times hymns are sung in community in choirs, a powerful shared experience both physically and vocally for the singers and the listeners. According to Merriam-Webster (n.d.), a hymn is a song of praise or joy, and its etymology is of Greek origin. One only needs to experience listening to a gospel choir or singing in one, to be infected by this joyous, optimistic, and soulful might almost by osmosis.

In Krystal's class, inspired by hymns, students are asked to compose an authentic written affirmation phrase. Here are a few examples that students have penned: *my music history class challenges me, and I want to reconnect to my love of music; I have a lot of anxiety about the art critique coming up, I wish I could make art more calmly and sleep all night; Asking me to use my voice in classes makes me shut down and be silent; I imagine myself being able to recite poems I write adding sounds.* Once the phrases are written down, read to the self, and then read aloud, the class collaborates to match a simple melody to each affirmation. We become a choir in this aforementioned sacred space and sing the affirmations one after another in an associative oratorio. Each affirmation then becomes part of a one-time opera that tells of both tragedy and joy; like all operas.

The Story That Objects Hold: Sacred Objects

Objects are so important that an entire psychological theory called object relations theory was developed based on observing how important objects were to babies, infants, and toddlers (Hamilton, 1999). In this book, we specifically focus on transitional objects, or tangible three-dimensional items that can bring us back to those moments in childhood that comforted us and made us feel safe and secure, as we moved from one place to another. We have outgrown our pacifiers, stuffies, and blankies, and we have moved on.

Many ancient cultures have used objects such as talismans and amulets for protection, fertility, and more in rituals and ceremonies. The reason we mention this here is that we have observed that our adult students and participants are also in need of transitional objects, and so are we.

In *The Amulets, Talismans, and Magical Jewelry: A Way to the Unseen, Ever-Present, Almighty God*, author Barbara Black Koltuv (2005) writes that people need to carry things with them, "We have fallen upon hard times. We are lost, beset, alone, and afraid. We need help... Amulets, talismans, and magical jewelry provide a beautiful, tangible bridge between us and the unseen..." (p. 3).

Objects of Transition

We have found that when our students are invited to bring objects to class, or photo images of objects, or to respond to objects we bring, then asked to write to those objects, about them, and from them, surprising words arise; some emotion-laden, some comical, some mysterious, all authentic. Some students connect and resonate with the religious and or spiritual aspects, of these as adult transitional objects, and some do not. We also believe that some adults, alongside the amulets and talisman, might still need some kind of soft, cuddly, huggable item; perhaps a pet, and it is OK!

People need to have a chance to write about why they are carrying these objects because they don't often recognize that they are carrying these objects with them, or what the reason is behind that. Perhaps it is a photograph: of their child, a beloved, a parent, or a place in their wallet; a piece of jewelry: an evil eye pin on their bag, a worry doll, or a worry stone in their coat pocket. It could be anything. Perhaps, simply something they were given by a person who is no longer with them, a stone they picked up on their hike, a sea shell, their guitar pick, a feather, a paintbrush, a spirit animal, a religious or cultural symbol, or their favorite perfume, it could be anything. We are tethered by these transitional objects to safer memories, places, and people. This is then symbolically transferred to us through these special items. Writing about what we need at the moment and turning that into a three-dimensional object that we can carry with us is something that we do when working with people who have experienced trauma, transition, or other life changes.

Objects That We Have Shared

Remember those glass jars filled with colorful individually wrapped hard candy that used to be on everyone's desks? Bankers, doctors, lawyers, teachers, the principal, the post office, and even sometimes at the dentist's office surprisingly. It was a sweet symbol to make you feel like you were at home. In Krystal's office, there is also a jar, but it does not have candy in it. Krystal's jar is full of miniature Mayan worry dolls, from Guatemala, that are made with tiny sticks wrapped with multi-colored thread. When a student arrives worried, upset, or anxious, Krystal might invite them to open the jar and choose one of these dolls to take home with them after the conversation to remember that there might be resilience, problem-solving, and comfort. Looking at the doll and holding it will be a symbolic reminder of possible inner strength in the face of a challenge.

Inspirational Objects

We have been inspired by many artists throughout our lives, which animates our teaching, clinical work, personal lives, and writing. We cannot name or discuss all of these inspirational artists, but we can give you a small taste. For example, Picasso built sculptures from everyday found objects. He used brooms, a tractor seat, and a bicycle handlebar to create a bull's head. We found Picasso's exhibit inspirational, in that he gave importance to objects that were left behind that he then transformed into compelling magically, thought-provoking, and emotionally evocative works of art (MoMA, 2008).

In our classes, therapy, workshops, and private lives we use an assemblage, a clustering together and placement of found objects and the writing about them to connect and deepen the relationship between the viewer, and the feelings, associations, and memories that these objects and their placements bring up.

The Turkish writer Orhan writes about how collecting objects is more than just hoarding or appreciating things. Pamuk passionately collects objects of desire; objects that remind him of a love affair that has ended. In *The New York Times* book review, Edmund de Waal (2021) writes that the storyteller in the book realizes that "objects beget narratives, just as stories need objects" (para, 1).

Objects do not have to be beautiful, perfect, eye-pleasing, new, calming, or aesthetically pleasing; they can be jarring, broken, dried up, cracked, crooked, and used. In other words, inspirational objects can connect us to the entire spectrum of human feelings, from whole to broken and everything in between. Objects carry all of our stories, from generations and ancestry of the past to this very moment in time. For this reason, we deeply believe in writing about objects as a transformative and therapeutic tool.

Writing Invitations

1 **Write Your Ode**

As a warm-up to this writing invitation, look at the writing implement you are writing with at this very moment: pen, pencil, phone, computer, or marker, perhaps. Write an ode to this instrument that is your writing tool, the object that allows you to write. Once you have done the first part, take a break. Reread the ode. See how you feel about it. Then, look for objects in your living space that invite odes, from the most seemingly mundane to the most story and memory-laden. This is not unlike a thank you note for the existence of the object.

2 **Nothing Is Mundane**

Perhaps we may consider things to be boring or mundane simply because we lack the time or ability to give our full attention to experiencing the dynamics of the THING. With this in mind, create a pause in your probably over-laden day and look around you with ease, care, and time; slow your looking down. When your eyes land on a THING that you **see daily**, focus on it from many directions, sideways, upside down, far away, very, very close up. Then put it down and write all the details you have noted and noticed without letting your pen leave the paper or fingers leave the computer. Read what you have written after 10 minutes. Is the THING still mundane? Is it not? Write about that too.

3 **Write Your Prayer**

Though many consider prayers to be pre-written for us in our diverse and rich faiths and spiritual beliefs, we invite you here to write an additional one yourself. If you prefer, think of this as making a wish. Think of a personal situation, yours or another's, in which a prayer could be said aloud, whispered, or said silently in one's heart. We believe that we all have been in situations in which we prayed for something. Perhaps for help or support or strength, perhaps patience, anything at all that comes up. Write the prayer down to whomever you want. Then, rewrite the words on a small piece of paper and add some ornamentation. Put this in your wallet, hang it on your bathroom mirror, or place it under your pillow. Anywhere that feels right. Revisit this exercise when needed.

4   **Object Assemblage; Build an Altar**
Seek out, explore, meander, and find objects that speak to you. Collect them, at one time or over time. Assemble on a tabletop indoors, outdoors, anywhere. Add to this at times. Write about how and what you have collected, honored, assembled, and put together in your own personal altar. It might even be an altar to writing! Write to it, about it, from it…

5   **Tell the Story of the Place Where One Has Lived: A Written Home Timeline**
Pretend that you have to write a description of all the homes that you have lived in from birth until now for a CV (curriculum vitae). Including ones that were for any amount of time. Get into the details of the homes, the countries, the cities, the neighborhoods, the streets, the neighbors, the home, the years, who you lived with, etc. Write this slowly, daily for a few weeks. Allow the senses and memories to arise. The scents, seasons, sounds, tastes, and scenes.

6   **Poetry Response**
Use Mary Oliver's poem "BONE" (2005) as a writing prompt to write your own poem about an object that you have found that has stimulated your curiosity, whetted your imagination's appetite, or responded directly to Oliver's words. Please find "BONE" (Oliver, 2005) online.

Resources

Songs

"This little light of mine" (song). (1920s).
    The composer and lyricist of this gentle song are unknown; however, it has been sung and performed by many artists in a variety of different genres including folk, blues, jazz, and country to name a few.

Poems

Any poetry by Mary Oliver. One of our favorites is "Storage." It was first published in 2015 in Felicity. The copyright is held from 2017 by NW Orchard LLC. You can find it on page 7 in the 2020 Penguin Books collection of her poems, *Devotions: The Selected Poems of Mary Oliver*.

Videos

To learn more about collectors and collecting, you can check out this, documentary from C. Hall titled "COLLECT – A documentary about collectors, collecting & collections" uploaded to YouTube on December 24, 2020. Here is a link: https://www.youtube.com/watch?v=qce-gYhLcpY

For a video focusing on book collecting, you can explore this title from the jessethereader YouTube channel, "A collection of books about books," uploaded on May 9, 2023. Here is a link: https://www.youtube.com/watch?v=neJT7A0dCmo

References

Black Koltuv, B. (2005). *Amulets, talismans, and magical jewelry: A way to the unseen, vverpresent, almighty God.* Nicolas-Hays Incorporated.

Bullock, W., Le Guin, U.K., & Shevelev, R. (1993). *The enchanted landscape: Photographs 1940–1975.* Aperture.

Carlyle, T. (1838). *The French revolution: A history* (Vol. 1). Charles C. Little and James Brown.

de Waal, E. (2012, November 13). Cultural artifacts. *The New York Times.* https://www.nytimes.com/2012/12/02/books/review/the-innocence-of-objects-by-orhan-pamuk.html

Hamilton, G.N. (1999). *Self and others: Object relations in theory and practice.* Rowman and Littlefield Publishers, Inc.

Merriam-Webster. (n.d.). Hymn. In *Merriam-Webster.com dictionary.* Retrieved December 16, 2023, from https://www.merriam-webster.com/dictionary/hymn

Museum of Modern Art (MoMA). (2008). *Focus: Picasso sculpture.* https://www.moma.org/calendar/exhibitions/100

Neruda, P. (1994). *Odes to common things* (Bilingual ed.). Bulfinch.

O'Donohue, J. (2000). *Eternal echoes: Celtic reflections on our yearning to belong* (Reprint ed.). Harper Perennial.

Oliver, M. (2005). *Why I wake early: New poems.* Beacon Press.

Tynianov, Y., & Shukman, A. (2003). The ode as an oratorical genre. *New Literary History, 34*(3), 565–596.

Chapter 4

Writing Details
The Spine of Soulful Writing

Krystal Leah Demaine and Tamar Reva Einstein

Welcome Mat: This chapter hones in on the details and development of expressive writing by bringing in mindfulness and somatosensory experience. Readers will learn about generating a writing inventory, cultivating mindful writing, nurturing natural writing, and exploring textural syntax in expressive writing. Details are often glanced over in our fast-paced world.

Delving into the Details

There is an idiom that says, *God is in the details*. This expression has been attributed to many people. Details bring to life stories that might otherwise be flat and difficult to connect to. When describing a dream, a memory, a photograph, a felt sense, a wish, or a trauma, the details are what enhance the experience. If we were referring to a photograph or an image on a computer, we would say the more pixels the better, the sharper the image.

In our writing classes, we ask people to look and write not only through their eyes but also through multiple senses. We suggest writing from the ears, from the skin, from the taste buds, through nostrils, and through the eyes. As Anaïs Nin (1976) wrote, "If you do not breathe through writing. If you do not cry out in writing, or sing in writing, then don't write, because our culture has no use for it" (p. 13). If you believe in it, one could imagine writing from your third eye, the part that connects to your soul, spirit, and heart. When written with such attention details can become profound. When we read a piece of writing, we want to know the details: what the fabric felt and smelled like, what time of the day it was, which direction the sun shone and the moon cast, what season it was, how the hair fell across a person's face, what they were wearing, what sensations were felt on the skin, what sounds were heard in the background, what emotions were experienced, and what were they thinking. It is the details that grab and hold the reader in the essence of the scene. Once we have magnified the details of what we have been paying attention to and we can write them down we are given a gift that now can be unwrapped. In the classes that we

DOI: 10.4324/9781003391876-5

teach and in therapy we unwrap this gift of description very slowly because it is multi-layered and fragile.

As humans, we don't often have the time to slow down and look at details in our lives. Life moves fast, and modern life is very oriented toward quantity and speed. In the past, letter writing required inserting a quill into an inkwell. Words were scribed with intent and the ink that generated those words required time to dry before the paper, sometimes scented paper, was folded over and placed in an envelope. The ink would smudge if it was not dry before the paper was folded. Nowadays, we send letters electronically, referred to as emails, which seem to travel faster than the speed of light, and sometimes because of the rushing we don't even proofread, let alone give time to let some ink dry. Details are the spine of mindful and soulful writing.

Writing in Nature: Playing in the Mud and the Crunching of the Leaves

Being in nature offers a buffet of sensory experiences without the white table-cloth. By leaving the four-wall sterile classroom and stepping into a space where nature reigns, we become as small as the tiny spider eggs we may find hanging miraculously in a handwoven sack between two twigs.

Krystal and her students go out to nature for some of their classes. This change of setting is done purposely to invite a more visceral experience that will be written about afterward. For one of the outings, she prepares the students by showing the film *Rivers and Tides: Andy Goldsworthy, Working with Time* (Von Donop & Riedelsheimer, 2001) and often uses Dr. Seuss's *The Lorax* (1971), quoting the main character who repeatedly says, "I speak for the trees," as a response to the trees being cut down (p. 14). Goldsworthy is an artist who goes to many places in nature and creates impermanent installations that both amplify the innate beauty out there and show the exquisite, magical, and gorgeous side of how nature is constantly changing. He is also telling a story between the lines, of deep respect, like the Lorax, of nature.

Krystal takes her students for a walk outside of the indoor classroom and out to nature, telling them ahead of time to focus on their awareness of what is around them while outside. Krystal and her students walk together in the autumn in New England when the leaves are colorful and the air is sweet and musty. At a certain point on the trail where there is a clearing, Krystal stops and asks the students to find a spot to sit that feels nice to them. She states that this will be their outdoor studio for the class meeting and points out perimeter boundaries of the space in which students can feel free to meander, while in the clearing.

Once her students find a place to sit, perhaps on a rock, tree stump, or the ground, Krystal asks her students to take out their journals and begin to write a list of all the colors they see, all the sounds they hear, all the sensations their body receives, what they imagine the leaves and trees taste like, and all of the scents they smell. They are asked to do this in total silence. When the writing part is done, Krystal asks students to stay in their chosen locations as she opens her card deck called, *Sacred Forest Cards*. She walks around to each student asking them to choose a card from the deck, hold it, look at it, and then draw a sketch of the card in their journal with a pencil and write about what association the card connects them to about being outdoors, writing, and sketching. Afterward, they all stand up in a circle and take turns sharing their cards and associative words. Krystal then asked the students to find a partner or small group of others based on whose word resonated with them. Once the partnerships are identified, Krystal gives the students 30 minutes to play and create in nature and only with natural objects. She further reminds the students to take care and be sensitive to not disturb the natural environment, reminding them of the work of Andy Goldsworthy (2001), whom they previously studied in their classroom, who believes that one should not impose oneself on nature but see it as your friend.

After the students finish creating in nature, they walk together as a large group to see the final constructions. Krystal has found it astounding to see what has been made by these groups. The students have built shelters and forts in which their bodies can fit, and miniature magical worlds that seem to have sprouted up from childhood fairytales, they also weave headpieces made of flowers and grasses. They create fragile installations that are reminiscent of spider webs made from sticks, feathers, and leaves. The nature installations are photographed so that the students have time outside of class to revisit the images and the experience and then write about the process and the product again. In an homage to Goldsworthy (2001), the students are reminded of how important it is to bond with the natural world through artmaking. Some of the after-effects of this outing that are highlighted in their writings are: how much they enjoyed playing in nature again, that they didn't get out to nature enough, and they didn't realize that nature could be their new studio space. This is interesting because Andy Goldsworthy usually makes all of his art outdoors turning nature into his studio space and friend; the students have now done the same.

Tamar connects writing in nature by asking the participants, second-year arts therapies master students in a three-day-intensive phototherapy course, to meander outdoors alone with their cameras. Meandering is a lost way of walking in our fast-paced and goal-oriented world. The camera can be a friend on this journey as it gently forces us to stop, pause, and look through the lens as we walk. Similar to the teaching of Thich Naht Hahn, who reminds us to slow down and even pause (Lattin, 1997). The space in which the students are asked to go outdoors is the gardens and paths of a small Jerusalem college; this provides for lots of hidden nooks and crannies and open space as well. 20 to 30 minutes are given to go out, walk slowly alone, camera in hand, looking in all directions including under things, and taking photographs. Upon returning to the classroom, the photos are moved to their laptops, to be seen in a larger format. They then review the photos, look at them with care, and write about themes, patterns, or stories that may arise. Then they take a break. After the break, they are asked to choose one photo that spoke to them the most, and they write again. They share aloud. Tamar then hands out tiny plastic frames from 35mm camera film negatives, once used for showing slides in the analog photo days, which she collected for years as photo shops were closing. The students are asked to move the frame around the image and find the most poignant place. Reframing the objects in their photos. Each time they find a possible poignant place they are asked to take a photograph of it and one photo is chosen at the end of the process. Tamar gives at least 20 minutes for this process. The classroom becomes full of exclamations like *"Wow," "Oh my God,"* and *"Look what I found,"* and sometimes there is body language changing, and tears rise or fall as well.

Then, the students are then asked to edit the photo digitally, only leaving the new reframed zoomed-in part. They write about this. Often personal, meaningful themes arise, which surprise the students, as an hour before these objects were not connected to them at all. Now, after writing, they take ownership.

To paraphrase what a student shared after this exercise, her photograph of a broken manhole under a blooming almond tree represented the story of her life over the past few months. She saw the danger in this, but also that the hole could be fixed. She was reminded that it was good to be aware of these holes in life and to try not to fall into them. The student also became aware of the juxtaposition of the sweet perfume of a pink blooming tree next to a sewage manhole. What a cathartic photo-induced process! The next day she showed Tamar that she had made art from the photo, written more, that the image had sent her on a deep journey, perhaps as deep as that manhole is.

Being out in nature, either in urban nature or in the country, is a great place to find writing inspiration. Nature has all, from growth in the dark, bulbs, and roots nourishing what grows above toward light from the depths to breaking branches, layers of leaves composting a new generation of shoots, all cycles of life from seed to death, like human growth from dark womb to life then back to the dark earth.

Ekphrastic Writing

For years, we have given participants photographs of artwork to describe in detail through writing. We continued to do this during the COVID-19 pandemic over Zoom. The process of writing about an image is an ancient Greek ritual known as "ekphrasis." Ekphrastic in Greek means honoring the piece of art. We were surprised that we hadn't known about this age-old writing ritual, somehow it had passed us by. We discovered it during the COVID-19 lockdown when we found *The Ekphrastic Review* (2023) online.

In our classes we ask students to look at an image of a famous painting, sculpture, or photograph and react to it through writing from both emotional and visual input and output. For example, on Zoom the very first day we had to teach during the pandemic in March 2020, Tamar, with the generous help of the university's IT squad as she had no idea what she was doing online, posted three photographs of artwork: one sculpture, one photograph, and one painting. The students were asked to choose one image that spoke to them the most, as we moved through this chaotic world paved in the unknown communally.

The students were asked to write 250 words about the image they chose. The writing was to be prompted by the photograph. The students were reminded to look at the photograph often while writing. They were asked to let words flow, feelings to lead them, to try to find a quiet place to engage in this process, which was very difficult to do while many people were all home together at the same time. We reminded them that it was fine to repeat words if it felt necessary, to not judge their grammar or care about the piece making sense to anyone else or even to themselves; just to sit alone looking at the image that they chose and to write. They were told that the image and writing would be discussed at the next meeting two weeks later. This would be the first-ever Zoom meeting that then became a much more familiar meeting space.

Once Tamar's class met on the shared online platform, together they viewed the three images, and almost all of the students shared their writing. It is not surprising that much of the writing had to do with the unknown, the surprise, and the fear that was rampant as the virus at the beginning of the pandemic, and the experience of what it had felt like to have an image to focus on during a time when no one understood the boundaries of this new time we were thrown into.

In response to the uncertainty of the pandemic, an associative image that arises for us, as we recall those days, is standing at the edge of the seashore and looking out realizing that there is an endless body of water in front of us, whose shoreline is amorphic and whose safe harbor is nowhere to be seen. Even a lighthouse was nowhere in sight. So, the writing and the sharing connected us—the authors as well as our students—all in little boxes to each other, to our writing, feelings, and fears, and the exercise served as a temporary safe haven as the tides changed and the water rose.

Details make writing spineful as opposed to spineless, and soulful as opposed to soulless. We all become braver with our words and safer in our sentences when we write in spaces and situations that are cushioned and contained both softly and in a trustworthy manner. Each tiny letter, word, sentence, and paragraph builds the soulful spine vertebrae by vertebrae into one's own upright story.

Writing Invitations

1   Writing on Stones

Go to nature and collect smooth stones, the smoothest you can find. Rivers and oceans can contain wonderfully smooth stones. Paint on the stones (acrylic is ideal) and then write words on the stones (we prefer paint pens or indelible markers like Sharpie). Write positive affirmations or single words on the stones that have meaning to you. Perhaps, you may place these stones in parts of your home, a pocket of a coat you don't wear often, or the outdoors near your home where you don't look often, surprise yourself!

2   **Fingerprints**

Fingerprints are unique for almost every person, and in some officialities, fingerprints are used for identification purposes. Take a look at your fingerprints, photograph them, draw the tiny details, press them into clay or sand to make an impression, or actually, press your fingers into an inkpad and print your fingerprints on paper. Allow yourself to view your fingerprint impression and see what patterns emerge. In detail write about the contours, the curves, the symbols, and the shapes, and make lists and notes. Write about the role, the history, and the journey of how your fingerprints make you who you are. Remember how magical it is that no two people in the world have the same fingerprints, which is quite outrageous if you think about it.

3   **Just a Taste**

For this invitation, please choose a small single piece of food that is small enough to hold in your hand. Some great options might include a nut like an almond or pistachio (in the shell is best), a berry, a cube of cheese, a cracker, or a piece of chocolate. Using your fingers, feel the food and write down its texture: smooth, bumpy, round, slimy, rough; using your eyes, write down the color, shape, and form; using your nose, write down all of the smell qualities you detect: sweet, bland, spicy; using your ears squish it, crack it open, break it, and listen to the quality of the sound. Lastly, put the food in your mouth and taste all of the qualities. Allow the sensory experience of the tiny piece of food to wash over you as you write down the full list of sensory qualities you experience with this tiny piece of food.

4   **Breath Mantra**

Zen master and spiritual leader Thich Nhat Hanh (2002) reminds his practitioners to silently say a prayer or mantra each time they breathe in and out.

To begin your practice, simply practice breathing in and breathing out. Write down what you are breathing in and what you are breathing out. You can practice as many times and with as many words as you would like. Keep your words and your practice simple. You can place your written breath mantra next to you as you sleep or keep it in your pocket as a reminder to breathe.

5   **Details in the Movements**

Observe yourself slowly moving through one simple task. Some examples include opening the lid on a container, combing your hair, turning on a light switch, or taking a single step. Observe your movements very slowly and exaggerate each teeny-tiny gesture.

List each micro-movement, from the blink of an eyelash to the bending of your knee, and number these steps, 1., 2., 3…. Sometimes it is helpful to listen to slow-tempo music as you move. From Krystal's experience, pieces of music, around 40–50 beats per minute are ideal. We may suggest for example

Beethoven's *Moonlight Sonata*, or become a DJ and search for music that you find soothing and slows you down. After you have written your list, write what you notice in your movements that you haven't noticed before once the movements were slowed down. What did you discover about the pace of your movements, the rhythm of your movements, and how paying attention to your movement affects you?

6   **Ekphrastic Writing with Photographs, Paintings, and Photos**
Ekphrastic writing celebrates and honors an image by writing about it; this exercise is an invitation to write in this ancient manner. Choose a favorite painting or photograph. Sit down across from the image and begin writing either a poem, a short story, or any other writing form that comes to you. Look at the image intermittently so as not to lose contact with what it offers. If you so choose, you can do this in a museum, art gallery, or your home. Notice if this writing has led you to surprises, to realizations, to a new way of looking at this image. Has free association led you down a new path? Are you sad, happy, angry? Write about that too.

Resources

Films

To learn more about Andy Goldsworthy, check out this 2001 film produced by A. Von Donop and directed by T. Riedelsheimer, *Rivers and Tides: Andy Goldsworthy, Working with Time*. It is from Mediopolis Film.

In addition to the book, Dr. Seuss's *The Lorax* was made into a film in 2012. Directed by C. Renaud for Illumination Entertainment and Universal Pictures.

Books

We mentioned both Mary Oliver and Thich Nhat Hahn in this chapter. We recommend Mary Oliver's *Devotions*, reprinted in 2010 by Penguin Books. Also from 2010, we recommend Nhat Hahn's *You Are Here: Discovering the Magic of the Present Moment* published by Shambhala.

Art

A great painting to inspire soulful writing is from K. Hokusai (1830–1832), *The Great Wave off Kanagawa*. Found at The Met, New York City, USA, you can learn more about it on their website: https://www.metmuseum.org/art/collection/search/45434.

For photography, we recommend exploring that from Ansel Adams. You can check his work out in person at the Ansel Adams Gallery in Yosemite National Park, California, USA, or on their website: https://www.anseladams.com/.

Places

There are many wonderful places to explore, below are three we recommend with links to their websites.

- Chinese Garden, Montreal (Canada): https://espacepourlavie.ca/en/chinese-garden
- The Strand Bookstore, New York City (USA): https://www.strandbooks.com/

The Rubin Museum of Art, New York City (USA): https://rubinmuseum.org/

References

Ekphrastic Review (2023). Home page. https://www.ekphrastic.net/

Hanh, T. N. (2002). *Present moment wonderful moment: Mindful Verses for daily living.* Parallax Press.

Lattin, D. (1997, October 12). Sunday interview - Stop running, start being. *San Francisco Chronicle.* https://www.sfgate.com/news/article/SUNDAY-INTERVIEW-Stop-Running-Start-Being-2801807.php

Nin, A. (1976). *In favor of the sensitive man and other essays.* Harcourt Brace Jovanovich.

Seuss, S. (1971). *The Lorax.* Random House.

Von Donop, A. (Producer), & Riedelsheimer, T. (Director). (2001). *Rivers and tides: Andy Goldsworthy, working with time* [Film]. Mediopolis Film.

Chapter 5

Writing and Metaphor
Stepping Away to Get Closer

Krystal Leah Demaine and Tamar Reva Einstein

Welcome Mat: This chapter engages creative writing in metaphor. Readers will explore themselves through a symbol to examine parts of the self, place of origin, and current place of space, season, and weather. Come join in this sea of words as we navigate with our pens and hearts as compasses.

Defining Metaphors in Writing

The great philosopher Aristotle once said "The greatest thing by far is to be a master of metaphor" (350 BCE/1994–2000, part 22). Metaphors use symbolism to describe an object or action using figures of speech that are not to be taken literally. In the introduction to his book *The Role of Metaphor in Art Therapy* (2007), seasoned art therapist Bruce Moon described the etymology of the word metaphor:

> The word metaphor is derived from the Greek *meta*, meaning above and beyond, and *phorein*, meaning to carry from one place to another; the latter is the same root of *amphora*, an ancient Greek vessel for carrying and storing precious liquids. Metaphors in language are also carriers: they hold information that hide meaning in symbolic form.
>
> (p. 3)

When we introduce metaphoric writing, we explore metaphors that are used in daily language to give examples of how metaphor is so prevalent. Oftentimes people don't realize how prevalent metaphors are in language, but as humans, it is very common to communicate with one another through metaphor. However, metaphors do not travel well between languages. They are indigenous to specific languages and can be impossible to translate. Yet because we also train therapists, we ask our students to think of metaphors that are used to describe emotions, or that they heard on the bus, or that they use and don't even realize they are using metaphor. For example, the following is a list of metaphors related to emotions:

I tripped myself up.
I am drowning in anxiety.

DOI: 10.4324/9781003391876-6

My family is a heavy burden on my shoulders.
I feel like I am sinking in quicksand.
My world is upside down.
You are such a couch potato.
She looked like a deer in headlights.
I am a rollercoaster of emotions.
You are the apple of my eye.
I am in the eye of the storm.
We are attached at the hip.
I am a cup of spilled coffee.
I wear my heart on my sleeve.
I want to move on to the next chapter of my life.
I am not in focus today.
I'm feeling overexposed.

The above metaphors of course are not to be taken literally; the gift of metaphor is that we understand what the phrase means. People can move away from their lived personal experiences, write them down in words or other art forms, and then like the amphora, save them like sacred oil that is moved from one place to another and can then be extracted and explored.

We use the term welcome mat as the first exposure to the writing of metaphors. You are wiping your feet and walking in. You are not inside yet. You haven't even rung the doorbell. You will enter the writing at your own pace, word by word, one step at a time.

What happens when the caterpillar goes into the chrysalis, turns into a gel, a liminal nothing, and then into a butterfly? Or what happens to the snake when they shed its skin? What is the metaphor that you go to in your writing? Tamar has often gone to metaphoric poetry at different points of her life that clarify rites of passage, grief, and even love stories. The below poem describes one of the examples of her writing on how painful life can seem as she moves through different stages and seasons of life. One can discern from the poem that Tamar is writing about herself.

"Growing Pains", a metaphor poem
by Tamar Einstein (1985, unpublished)

The snake,
In its last phase of shedding,
Discarding its now outgrown skin,
experiences great discomfort.

The eyes,
Once piercing,

Are now filmy lenses,
Through which all images,
Dark and light,
Are blurred.

The skin,
Once breathtakingly beautiful,
In both pattern and hue,
Is now a milky distorted coat of arms.
Unclear and uninviting.

The snake,
In its last phase of shedding,
Discarding,
Disrobing,
Once swift on its smooth belly,
Moves only to disengage the newborn gloss,
From the peeling skin,
Once home to its body.

In blindness, it lies,
Immobile in growing pains
Once finally shed,
The brittle skin shell is there to see,
To delicately touch.
An iridescent crackly shadow,
Of an outgrown shelter,
Of a growing pain,
In a cycle of growth.

The snake may not seem longer,
Or wider,
But the snake has grown through pain,
To painstaking beauty.

Metaphor in Teaching

When teaching phototherapy, Tamar often asks students to go out and photograph a tree. The tree can be old, new, whole, broken, in any season, in any place, and if they have such a photo that they took in the past it is fine to bring that one in as well. The images are brought on A4, printer-size paper, in black and white. The stories about the photos are told, including when, where, and how they decided to take that particular picture and what connects them to it now.

This round ends with all of the trees being laid out on the big table to look at more closely. After a short break, Tamar asks them to look at their photo again and to write what emotions it brings up, and how they feel similar or different from that tree; to pay attention to textures, directions, roots exposed or hidden, the frame, the closeness or distance, and the placement of the tree on the page. Is it front and center? Is it hidden amongst other trees? Is it partially out of the frame of the photo, perhaps out of focus?

The students' writings are then shared by those who choose. Often, autobiographical stories emerge from this metaphoric exercise. Folks are astonished at how they discover important self-reflective information from this writing. Some choose to take Tamar up on the invitation to take a photo of a tree once a day or once a week and write about it. These are often included in their end-of-the-year papers.

Using Metaphors in Therapeutic Writing

Metaphors and figurative language help therapy clients express their stories symbolically (Shkembi & Treska, 2023). Psychotherapist Virginia Satir (1988), best known for her seminal work in family therapy, created a theory called the Satir Iceberg metaphor (Innes, 2002) describing the seen and the unseen in what a person represents of their self. As Satir (1988) noted, "Family life is something like an iceberg: most people are aware of only about one-tenth of what is going on—the tenth that they can see and hear" (p. 17). The authors imagine this theory based on the fact that icebergs are mostly immersed in frozen water and humans only get to see the tip of them.

These examples reaffirm the power of metaphor used by other disciplines and not just expressive arts therapists, teachers, and supervisors. Metaphor is ancient and continues to be utilized as a tool in many helping professional's toolboxes. Lakoff and Johnson (1980) show how important metaphors are, stating that, "human *thought processes* are largely metaphoric" (p. 6). One might agree or disagree with this, but metaphors are very user-friendly and accessible when playing with words and phrases in writing; like a walk in the park, or a piece of cake.

Identity, Ancestry, and Writing: Using Metaphors to Tell Our Stories; Written Self-Portraits

Metaphors are a welcoming tool when writing about biographic or autobiographic memories and/or associations. When we feel that the timing is right to work on this topic with our students, which is usually when we know them quite well, the stories people carry within them are quite intimate and layered. We address this topic almost as if the participants and the group leaders are archeologists arriving at a new archeological dig site. One must be able to unearth the past while using tools that do not shatter or break what is found along the way.

The writing and the prompts should be gradual, and gentle, and honor the fragility of the ancient artifacts that make up people's lives. The idea of searching for a hidden treasure that you know is there can be daunting, both metaphorically and literally. It might be wise to use a tiny brush as you nudge away one layer of earth at a time. This can be a long and complicated process; one that is worth doing to reach your soul's awaiting hidden mysteries.

Students and participants might choose to research their identities, cultures, ancestry, and histories through diverse metaphors. This often begins with an arts-based experience that moves into a written piece. These metaphors can be as obvious as objects one has received from family members that have traveled through decades within their families to an abandoned partially burned-down house they drive by every day on their way to work; the choices are endless. To enhance attunement to one's past connecting to the senses may conjure pre-verbal memories of where one is from (Kossak, 2015).

We present a list of actual objects that we have used over the years to connect people to their personal and collective histories and parts of the self to ignite the imagination by focusing on a metaphoric symbol. Remembering that metaphor simultaneously allows one to move away from something to get closer to it.

- Self as an ancient vessel (that might be cracked, broken, repaired, or restored)
- Self as a flower growing from a bulb, seed, root, or rhizome (root rot, growing in the dark, composted, weather exposure, or transplanted)
- Self as a meal (ingredients, recipe, flavors, manner of serving, or persona of the chef)
- Self as a mountain (hills, rocky, icy, desert, plateau, or volcanic)
- Self as a body of water (lake, river, stream, ocean, swamp, or bog)
- Self as a machine (washing machine, vehicle, vending machine, ATM, flashlight, or food processor)
- Self as a building (place of worship, a gym, a factory, a school, a historical library, a public garage, a convenience store, or a home)
- Self as a holiday (shopping, food, attire, rituals, location, or travel)
- Self as a book (pages, words, illustrations, location, typed or handwritten, inscriptions, musty, binding, or cover)
- Self as a language (accent, mother tongue, forgotten languages, spoken versus written, or body language)
- Self as a place on the map (location, size of land, what or who is on the land, where am I and how did my ancestors get here, by choice or not, by boat, plane, on foot, running away from or toward)

A Metaphor for the Self

In Krystal's classroom, she uses the tree as a metaphor for students to explore the self. To begin piquing the senses. Before the students arrive, Krystal prepares the space by pinning images of all different kinds of trees around the classroom walls: evergreens, maple, oak, fruit, flowering, willow, and palms. She fills the room with audio sounds from nature and sprays a light scent of pine and fruit essential oils in the air. She invites her students to a circle where yoga mats are placed in a circle, fanned out from the center of the room. She places a packet of individually wrapped airdry clay, a wooden stick, and a piece of black scratch paper on each mat. She asks each student to sit or lay on a mat of their choosing with their journals, and notice the sounds, images, and smells in the room. Once everyone is on their mat, Krystal guides the students through a short visualization imagining their body as a tree with roots (long, straight, curled, deep), a trunk (narrow, weathered, carved in, wide), and branches (long, curvy, arched, bowed, leafy, fruity, nutty). She asks the students to stretch their arms like branches growing from the floor until everyone is in an upright seated position. Once everyone is seated, she asks the students to pick up their airdry clay, open the packaging, hold the clay in their hand, and create a natural form; allowing the clay to mold naturally, without effort, but with intention and care. She tells the group that this clay will symbolize the fruit, nuts, or seeds from the tree.

Once everyone has finished creating a clay form, Krystal asks the students to place the new object in front of them, draw a quick sketch of the object in their journal, and then write words to describe the object, being very objective. She then asks the students in a technique of backward chaining, based on the Kodaly method (Chosky, 1999) of teaching music dynamically, to write about the branches and the places that the object (fruit, seed, or leaf) grew from. She then asks the students to write a description of the tree trunk and then the tree roots in the same fashion.

Once each student has written their descriptions of the tree, she asks the students to pick up the black scratchy paper and wooden stick on their mat and to draw an image of the tree in their mind's eye by scratching away the black ink from the paper using the stick. As the students scratch on the paper, the black ink lifts away leaving color where they scratched. Once the students finish drawing their tree design, they are asked to return to their journals and write about what the colors revealed to them about their tree; and to dig deep and use their imaginations as they write. This act of revealing by scratching is very different from drawing on paper.

While the students write, Krystal places more art materials in the center of the room including glue, plastic gemstones, acrylic paint, various-sized paint brushes, boxes of oil pastels, and tissue paper. She then places a piece of 11″ × 14″ Bristol board or another kind of painting paper in front of each student on their mat. Once the students finish their writing, she asks them to look at the writing and their object and view it silently. She then asks the students to choose art supplies from the center of the room and make a visual reflection of themself as a tree using the materials on the piece of Bristol board paper. Once the visual art is finished, students are asked to write about what they see in the painting, starting very objectively and then moving into more figurative phrases, thoughts, feelings, and emotions. From all of the art and writing, students write a longer reflective poem or narrative that they share with their classmates in response to self as a tree.

While the sense of smell is not often used in expressive arts therapy in our experience, Tamar has brought this sense in as a way for students and participants to create and then write about their ancestral, historical, and cultural roots. The participants are asked to bring in spices, ground, and whole, which are part of their family traditions. Some bring coffee and tea bags, too. Then they are asked to use these spices to create a piece of art that tells the story of who they are and where they are from. The spices, Tamar explains, can be glued, built with, smushed into clay, turned into paint with water, glazed with clear glues, embroidered onto the fabric, and whatever other way seems right in the process. The room becomes an olfactory cacophony, windows are opened... The writing comes after a break when all have completed the artmaking, deep emotions arise at this point. Students discover surprising memories and family lore that bring up hidden feelings. There might be tears, anger, and joy. The sharing is authentic, moving, and carries the scents of the stories. It is an experience of making sense through scents.

Exploring the Name: What's Your Name?

"That which we call a rose by any other name would smell just as sweet," wrote William Shakespeare in Act 2, scene 2, in his play, *Romeo and Juliet* (ca. 1594). We have thought that in this quote, which Juliet famously says to herself, but is overheard by Romeo, referring to the feud between their families, who are from different social standings, Juliet means that no matter what his name would be she would still have the same feelings. That his name is meaningless to her in their shared story. Even today in certain cultures, communities, tribes, and families, men and women are forbidden to marry other men and women from specific families who share ancestral disagreements. Meaning, they do not want their last name to be carried on by that particular person. We have found in our experiences that names, nicknames, and family names can be important to our participants and clients. As Salman Rushdie wrote, "Names, once they are in common use, quickly become mere sounds, their etymology being buried, like so many of the earth's marvels, beneath the dust of habit." (*The Satanic Verses: A Novel*, 1988, p. 224). Your name has to do with your identity, ancestry, history, gender, belonging, how you are referred to, and how you refer to yourself.

On a more personal note, our names have specific meanings. Tamar, in Hebrew, refers to the date palm tree and its fruit the date. Her name was infrequently used both in her childhood in New York and afterward in Jerusalem, she was and still is referred to as Tammy. As Tamar ages, she has taken photographs of palm trees at different stages of development and seasons as an autobiographic arts-based inquiry. Krystal's first name comes from the ancient Greek word krystallos and means "ice." It refers to a variety of crystal gemstones, from emeralds to diamonds. So, we are both connected to nature by our names.

Our last names carry meanings as well. Einstein immediately brings up associations of the famous scientist and in Israel a favorite singer, but in the etymology of the word according to Jones (2008), it means "place encompassed by a stone wall" (p. 26). Einstein can also mean *one stone* in German. Her last name was the butt of many jokes and comments and still is. Teachers in particular loved reminding her how terrible she was at math with such an important name. Demaine has more than one meaning found online: an island that surrounds a home used by an owner, and inherited from Old French *demain*, from Late Latin *dē māne* ("early in the morning"), from Latin *dē* + *māne*, and from Proto-Indo-European **meh$_2$-* ("to mature, ripen") (Etymology online). We find it interesting that both of our names, Demaine and Einstein, refer to land. Krystal's last name had another layer to her story.

As Krystal described in her seminal book, *The Roots and Rhythm of the Heart* (2022), her given name Bloom was changed to Demaine by her paternal grandparents in 1940, the same year they married. The new name also trickled to her great grandparents, great aunts, and uncles, who also adopted the new identity. The name was chosen by her paternal grandmother, a poet and painter who adored French language and culture. Due to her grandmother's college education and sophistication in the arts, her name suggestion was respected and embraced. The family's rationale for changing the name was to hide their Jewish identity. This was different from people who were given new names for other reasons. For example, some people who got off the boat at Ellis Island in New York City were assigned a new name and enslaved people were given names.

Our Students' Names

In our classes, one of the first things expected is for students to say their names, to introduce themselves. Tamar usually begins by saying that the name introduction ritual will wait and first, there will be an arts-based writing-based experiential. To begin the activity, they are asked to write their names at the top of a page, lengthwise; they can choose their first name or surname. Then they are asked to associatively write a list of words under each letter. In the next step, they are asked to circle a few words that stick out to them as they reread the words. Then, they are asked to write a sentence, short paragraph, or poem using these words and adding whatever other words they want and need. Next, they read the pieces aloud, and say their names. After this, they circle a meaningful sentence. The final product of this process is that one by one they read their sentences aloud, as one student writes them down; a group poem is created. It is read aloud. This is a meaningful way to get to know one another and begin to feel connected. They are sent the poem by the scribe and asked to create art to bring to the next class.

We also want to mention names that might carry stories that the students do not want to use in class. Sometimes a student prefers a nickname, or a different name than the one that appears on our roster.

Regarding names and what they carry, Tamar once led a group, in which a participant was named Massada. The student spoke about how carrying the tragic biblical story of this desert mountain had a powerful effect on her, and at times she thought of changing her name but was afraid of insulting her parents. Some Orthodox Jews believe in going to a rabbi to change their names when they are sick, have done *Tshuva* (become more orthodox), or have not conceived a child. It is believed by some that by receiving a new name their luck will change.

The Giving Tree: Reading and Metaphor

One of the ways that Tamar warms the students up to metaphoric writing is by reading a children's book aloud. Often, she chooses *The Giving Tree* (Silverstein, 2002). This book allows for many emotions to arise, revelations of identification to resonate, and personal memories to come to the surface. Partially, this is due to the simple, but beautifully rendered line-drawing illustrations, and a storyline that is brilliant, complex, and easy to understand. After the story is read aloud, the students are asked to immediately draw a tree that is in some way related to the story and to their own life stories. They are then asked to sit in front of the art and write free-form sentences, stories, or whatever comes up in words. When the sharing begins the students are surprised by how they were able to connect deeply with intimate inner memories through a story that was not theirs. Once again, the gift of metaphor is experienced: moving away to get closer. A choreography in which all dancers can be both the audience and the performers. Witnessing from the outside and the inside; forming a ballet of the self and soul. Or putting their life stories in that Greek amphora, rare essential words like oils, that can be carried and moved with care to pour them out slowly and explore, imbibe through the pores of their spirits and souls. Then write as the word and the oil nourish their skin and stories.

Writing Invitations

1   **Photographs of Stepping Stones or Stumbling Blocks**
    You are invited to choose a photo of a path of stones from the internet, that you find in a book or magazine, or that you have taken. They might be stones over bodies of water, slippery, flat stones semi-sunk into earth leading into a forest, stone path bridges with wooden rails for support, or stone steps that lead to an endless horizon, for example. Look at the image, and ask yourself: Where am I on this path? What is this path? Over what does this path follow: Wild waters? Calm seas? Mud? Soft grass? Broken glass?... Write your answers down. Then, look again and ask yourself: How do I proceed or not proceed?

Write about the path: Did it feel safe, welcoming, mysterious, and/or familiar? What does walking on these stones feel like: Are they stepping stones, stumbling rocks, or both? Write again. After, add drawing, collage, writing, music soundtrack, or a movement choreography to the image. You can make your art manually and/or digitally in order to explore your journey more deeply.

2 **Self as Metaphor**

Use this list of questions as writing prompts. Write associative words, sentences, stories, prose, and poems with these and your imagination as your compass; you may choose to create art to illustrate your wordplay:

- Self as an ancient vessel (that might be cracked, broken, repaired, or restored)
- Self as a flower growing from a bulb, seed, root, or rhizome (root rot, growing in the dark, composted, weather exposure, or transplanted)
- Self as a meal (ingredients, recipe, flavors manner of serving, or persona of the chef)
- Self as a mountain (hills, rocky, icy, desert, plateau, or volcanic)
- Self as a body of water (lake, river, stream, ocean, swamp, or bog)
- Self as a machine (washing machine, vehicle, vending machine, ATM, flashlight, or food processor)
- Self as a building (place of worship, a gym, a factory, a school, an historical library, a public garage, a convenience store, or a home)
- Self as a holiday (shopping, food, attire, rituals, location, or travel)
- Self as a book (pages, words, illustrations, location, typed or handwritten, inscriptions, binding, or cover)
- Self as a language (accent, mother tongue, forgotten languages, spoken versus written, or body language)
- Self as a place on the map (location, size of land, what or who is on the land, where am I and how did my ancestors get here, by choice or not, by boat, plane, on foot, running away from or toward)

3 **Opposites**

Write about the following words with word associations. Once you have written, reread your writing and see if these in any way connect to inner opposing feelings metaphorically and/or literally, beliefs and or thoughts you might have. Write about that!

- Ugly cigarette butts and flowers
- Hot and cold weather
- Peace and war
- Health and sickness
- Soft and hard
- Angels and monsters
- I forget and I remember

4 Goals and Obstacles

Materials: gather glue and different kinds of paper. The paper may include newspapers, magazines, colorful paper, tissue paper, or something different. Tear the paper into smaller pieces and a variety of different sizes. Leave two untorn pieces of paper. On the back of one of the untorn papers, write the word *goals* and on the back of the other paper write the word, *obstacles*. On the empty side of the paper begin to place the torn pieces and then glue the torn pieces of paper building two abstract images: one of your goals and another image of obstacles. Once the collages are complete, look at them and write about the differences and similarities, the shapes that emerged, the forms, the colors, the amount of paper you used, and anything else that seems interesting. Use these collages as a visual metaphor for your goals and obstacles. Take time away from these images and look again a few days later. Write down anything you notice that you didn't notice the first time. After you write, you might feel moved to tear some of the words you have written and create a new collage.

Resources

Talks

In this July 4, 2011, discussion from the University of Oxford Podcast, James Grant, Lecturer in Philosophy at the University of Oxford shares his thoughts on, "Metaphor and Art". You can listen to it here: https://podcasts.ox.ac.uk/4-metaphor-and-art.

In her September 2012 TED-ED talk, *The Art of Metaphor*, Jane Hirshfield examines metaphor. You can watch it here: https://www.ted.com/talks/jane_hirshfield_the_art_of_the_metaphor?language=en.

Films

Far from the Tree (2017) reflects on Andrew Solomon's (2012, Schribner) book of the same title which discusses parents and their children, expectations, and identity. The documentary film is directed by Rachel Dretzin for Sundance Selects.

Books

This compelling 2007 book, *The Jewish Americans: Three Centuries of Jewish Voices in America*, by Beth Wenger discusses what it was like for Jewish Americans, and many who became famous when they first came to America. It is published by Doubleday Books.

Gender in Judaism and Islam: Common Lives, Uncommon Heritage, is an edited volume, feminist theory-oriented, and discusses the similarities and differences between Islam and Judaism when it comes to Gender. Published in 2014, it is edited by Firoozeh Kashani-Sabet and Beth Wenger for NYU Press.

Television Show

To see fascinating explorations of family history and learn about one's ancestry, watch *Finding your Roots with Henry Louis Gates Jr.* on PBS. Learn more on their website:
https://www.pbs.org/show/finding-your-roots.

Places to Go

To learn more about the history of immigration in the USA, visit Ellis Island in New York City. You can learn more about the museum there on their website: https://www.statueofliberty.org/ellis-island/.

Newsletters

For more exploration of metaphor from Jane Hirshfield, check out this July 7, 2021, article on *The Mariginalian* by Maria Popova, "The handle on the door to a new world: Poet Jane Hirschfield on the Magic and Power of Metaphor, animated". You can find it at this link: https://www.themarginalian.org/2021/07/07/jane-hirshfield-metaphor/.

References

Aristotle. (350 BCE/1994–2000). *Poetics.* S. H. Butcher (Trans.). Internet Classics Archive. https://classics.mit.edu/Aristotle/poetics.mb.txt

Chosky, L. (1999). *The Kodaly method I: Comprehensive music education volume 1.* Prentice Hall.

Demaine, K. (2022). *The roots and rhythm of the heart: Our musical connection to identity, sprit, and lineage.* Lightning Source.

Innes, M. (2002). Satir's therapeutically oriented educational process: A critical appreciation. *Contemporary Family Therapy, 24*(1), 35–56.

Jones, G.F. (2008). *German-American names.* Genealogical.com.

Lakoff, G., & Johnson, M. (1980). *Metaphors we live by.* University of Chicago Press.

Kossak, M. (2015). *Attunement in expressive arts therapy: Toward an understanding of embodied empathy.* Charles C. Thomas, Publishers Ltd.

Moon, B. (2007). *The role of metaphor in art therapy: Theory, method, and experience.* Charles C. Thomas Publisher, Ltd.

Rushdie, S. (1988/2008). *The satanic verses* (Reprint ed.). Random House.

Satir, V. (1988). *The new peoplemaking* (2nd ed.). Science and Behavior Books.

Shkëmbi, F., & Treska, V. (2023). Metaphor as a technique in therapy. *European Journal of Social Science Education and Research, 10*(1s), 39–48.

Silverstien, S. (2002). *The giving tree.* Harper Collins.

Chapter 6

The Children's Department

Childhood, Children's Literature, and Striving to Write More Like Children

Krystal Leah Demaine and Tamar Reva Einstein

Welcome Mat: This chapter discusses childhood and how children's literature and illustrations can be informed by dreams, memories, and creative and expressive writing concepts. The authors will explore the use of childhood experiences in writing and reflecting, recounting their own childhoods, and the use of children's literature in the clinical training of therapists in academia.

In this chapter, we would like to connect to childhood and children's books, as they pertain to writing. By this, we mean we both use childhood memories, books, and stories in groups as writing invitations and to open doors to the past that connect to the here and now. We invite you to join us in the playscape of curiosity and wonder in used bookstores, libraries, and old abandoned books. We consider all kinds of books: those you read to yourself, those that were read to you, and those that you may read to others. We'd also like to discuss the rekindling of curiosity for books you haven't read in a while.

A book can be an old friend you can revisit, perhaps someone you haven't seen in a while. It can also be something sacred, or something that conjures memories, perhaps untethered reminders from the past. Books can take us to new destinations and come with us on vacations, bus rides, to work, waiting rooms in doctor's offices, hospital situations, supermarkets, coffee shops, and perhaps many other places and situations in which you feel the need to run away and run toward your imagination even momentarily. Books can be a distraction from our lives, on all levels of the emotional spectrum; they can nourish, enrich, affirm, validate, and perhaps leave us with questions. Book transport us. We invite you into the world of children's books … and as Garrison Keillor wrote, "A book is a gift you can open again and again" (Lederer, 1991, p. 149).

Books, Bookshelves, Libraries, and Bookstores

We both grew up in homes filled with books: Tamar in an apartment in New York City and Krystal in a house in Rockport, Massachusetts. The books filled shelves: children's books, adult books, *MAD* magazines, and *Highlights* for children magazines, among other monthly or weekly journals, and newspaper

DOI: 10.4324/9781003391876-7

clippings. Some books were more accessible to us because of our height as children and some less so; but somehow, at least for Tamar, she tried to read them all. Both of us were read to by our parents, both before bed and at other times, and we both read to our younger siblings. Books were given as birthday and holiday gifts, and they were treasured. We continue these fond memories now with our own children and other children with whom we are connected. We also purchase and give children's books to adults we know.

When Krystal was young, she would visit the magical Toad Hall Bookstore, a tiny three-floor shop in Rockport, Massachusetts, built with granite stone and centered with a spiral staircase made of iron. The shop had a smell of new books with a rich aroma of fresh paper, ink, and leather binding, which struck Krystal each time she opened the wide antique oak door of the shop, which left her breathless by its heavy weight. When Krystal went to this bookstore, she made a direct descent down the spiral staircase to the children's room on the lower level; a small room, equally sized to the two floors above, only the children's room was filled with bean bags chairs, stuffed animals, twinkle lights, and garlands of children's storybook characters made in felt; and shelves filled with books just for children, setting the perfect magical spot for cozy and peaceful reading; akin to a book-filled forest in a fairy tale.

It is important to us to begin this chapter by sharing that we believe we would not have written this book if we had not been so exposed to and enamored with books starting at a very young age. From nursery school onward, books, the book corner, and storytelling time became another important part of our love of books. This led to being allowed to visit our school library at a very young age and then, excitingly, to get a library card and be able to browse the endless shelves and choose two books a week to take home. In the school library, at the librarian's desk, on the big, wooden, hardly reachable desk top, we would place our chosen books. The librarian would remove the library card from a small manila envelope pasted on the front page of the book and stamp it with the due date. We also had to sign our name on the little card on a line next to the date. A history of anyone who had ever taken the book out was written on those cards. We both loved looking at the handwritten names of those who had taken out the book before us. If and when there was a book, we wanted that we couldn't find, we were sent to the wooden brass-handled card catalogs, in which there was a little typed index card (typed on a typewriter) for every book in the library with information on that book including the code to where it could be found. The librarian would help us find which shelf and which section the book was located in, as it was organized using the Dewy Decimal system. One always hoped that no one had taken the book out. For Krystal, when she preferred going to the library rather than hanging out with her friends outdoors, she immediately headed for the magazine room where her favorite reading materials were nature magazines, all encased in hard plastic sleeves so the pages would not become tattered. They were treated with great care, remember this is before the digital age—there was only one copy of the magazine, you couldn't just get another one. Krystal also was enamored by the newspapers that were attached to long wooden dowels and were hung from racks. One could gently pull the newspaper off the rack as if you were taking down your laundry.

Both of us were very different in our reading habits. Tamar would have preferred to read the newspaper from the rack, whereas Krystal would have preferred someone else to read it to her. We were both bookworms in different ways.

By the time Tamar was in the fifth grade, she had read all of the books in her school library; she was a voracious reader and because of that, during reading period in class, she was sent downstairs to the kindergarten to read stories to the younger children, which she loved.

Alongside libraries, both Krystal and Tamar were taken to bookshops by their parents, yet another treasure trove of penned gifts. Both of us continue to love bookstores, especially used bookshops. Our love of books also means that every once in a while, we need to pare down the amount of books that we own—it's not that we're hoarding, we're just collecting, remember that!

Some of the books we have collected we have read and re-read while others are still waiting patiently for us. How many people do you know, including yourself that have piles of books next to their beds that they intend to read at some point in time? According to an article in *Big Think*, the Japanese have a special term for this, *tsundoku*, which is a practice of surrounding oneself with books that may never be read (Dickinson, 2018/2022). In the article, statistician Nassim Nicholas Taleb said that "surrounding ourselves with unread books enriches our lives as they remind us of all we don't know" (para 1). In other words, we agree that surrounding ourselves with books reminds us that we have more to learn. Every closed book can open new worlds once the first page is turned.

We are also very aware that there are people who cannot afford to buy books, who have not been so exposed to books, and who have not had books read to them before they go to sleep or at all. Books are not available to all children or adults globally, and some books are banned.

When Tamar visits the United States, she always goes to the Morgan Library in New York City as one of her pilgrimage stops. Tamar finds it calming to be in a library of ancient books that reach from the floor to the ceiling. The authors have visited bookshops together on their visits with one another.

Reading Out Loud and Being Read To

Throughout the years that we have taught, supervised, and led groups, we have noticed that adults enjoy being read to as much as children, as they also enjoy reading their written pieces aloud. Part of being read to and reading out loud is the feeling, sound, and rhythm of the pages being turned. This visceral aspect of reading a book or having a book being read to us is something that one cannot experience when reading from a screen of any sort.

When someone is read to, they are almost being given a gift; they are receiving words, a story, and perhaps illustrations while they do not have to think about anything else. The story reader might also feel while reading aloud that there is a special connection occurring between the person giving the story and receiving the story. The reader might become playful, use different words, sing songs, speak with accents or made-up voices, stop at certain places to ask questions, and allow the person listening to the story to make up their own sounds and words. This interpersonal experience is magical, leaves an imprint on both people and can build closeness page by page. It is unusual for adults to read a book to themselves out loud though very normal to read a book to a child out loud. This was brought to our attention by Krystal's nine-year-old son, Ezra, who asked Krystal if she ever read the book that she wrote out loud from beginning to end. This led to a conversation about audiobooks and how some people enjoy listening to long "grown-up books." We wonder if audiobooks are the adult version of being read to. Something to ponder…

When Krystal was young, she and her two little sisters would pile into her bed, in their pajamas, about 20 minutes before bedtime to listen to their dad read a bedtime story. Almost every night he read to his daughters from a very thick fairy tale and poetry book, which seemed to be 1,000 pages long to young children. As the tales and poems became familiar to the girls, they learned to memorize them by heart. On some occasions, Krystal's dad would improvise the stories, changing them to create new and imaginative endings. Tamar was read to by many different people as a young child, but when it was bedtime for her son, lights off, she would lie down in the bed next to him in the dark and make up a new story before he fell asleep. The going-to-sleep ritual was this making up of a new story. Tamar also read books to her son, but he loved the makeup stories.

According to Sheldon-Dean, writing for the Child Mind Institute, exposure to words helps children develop language and cognitive skills (Sheldon-Dean, 2023). Children who are exposed to reading every day have more expansive vocabularies and will have greater comprehension of books they will read in the future. Stories help children learn to be more empathetic and problem-solving. We believe that reading offers a multi-sensory experience, turning the pages, feeling the paper, hearing the sounds, and seeing the words all at once engages the brain, especially when you are being read to by a loved one where bonding is simultaneously occurring.

Curiosity and Writing: Reconnecting to Imagination and Creativity

We strive to write and teach writing to our students and participants in a way that invites them to use their writing and imagination like children. Meaning, that we direct ourselves and our participants to reconnect to their childhoods when play and curiosity were the engines that drove them to explore, express, and learn. These engines for some adults have become rusty and we intend to slowly remove the rust. We say to our students in the first week of the class,

> You might want to visit the hardware store and buy some rust remover for these studies because you will find that removing the rust from your imagination will be very helpful to your journey both when you study and when you are a therapist.

Once the rust is removed, which can take a couple of years, it might also be prudent to oil that engine regularly. Our prescription is the arts: the perfect lubricant for a rusty engine or imagination.

The reason we begin the academic year with our expressive arts therapy students discussing rust removal is that children naturally learn through exploring and curiosity; from covering themselves with apple sauce to playing with a half-full bottle of water for an hour, or a pile of stones and telling incredibly detailed stories as they do so. "If given free rein to paint, to sing, to dance, to play, to experiment with language and to dramatize, children will do so spontaneously" (Landy, 1993, p. 360). Take a moment to watch a child playing and perhaps this will be clearer to you. Children are natural storytellers. As children get older, they then move this experimentation, dramatization, and spontaneity to their writing. If invited to do so, creating art and creative writing is how adults play.

Our personal experience studying with McNiff, one of our beloved mentors, over decades, has left us with a spine of imagination, a heart of curiosity, and a soul of playfulness. All of these creative elements are interconnected by veins in which art flows. As McNiff (2003) wrote, "Creativity can be defined as an original act of imagination that brings something into existence. It is a desire and innate drive to make new connections between things, to give form, and to transform" (p. 235). According to Etymonline (n.d.), the etymology of the word *curiosity* includes a desire to know or learn to be inquisitive, meddlesome, and inquiring eagerly, as well as a desire to know or learn what is strange or unknown. In Latin, the word *curiosity* is also "akin to *cura* care" (para 2). We find it fascinating that the word care is connected by its ancient Latin roots to the word, curious. Writing allows us to pay attention to our curiosity level. Curiosity invites us to touch details, play with the unknown, smell strangeness, and inquire through play and dramatization.

Tamar has heard many writing teachers say that the more you read the better you write. Better in this book means authentic. We are not discussing what is most publishable, highly regarded by critics, accessible, and realistic to most people; we are referring to writing that comes from the heart and soul. To us, that is the "better" stuff. Therefore, when writing, although you are an adult, we welcome you to reconnect or newly connect to words and writing through your imagination, playfulness, inner forgotten artist, playwright, storyteller, songwriter, poet, graffiti artist, puppeteer, or actor; in the same manner that children, naturally, freely, intuitively play with words and stories, in the same way they play with toys.

Roslyn Petelin (2022), author of *How Writing Works* says that "reading and writing are intimately connected in an osmotic relationship" (p. 11). If we want to learn to write well, we need to engage in reading regularly. Reading helps improve our sentence structure, spelling, word choice, rhythm, and punctuation. Petelin further suggests reading widely on broad and diverse topics, taking notes, and thinking about what you read. We would like to add that being around books, bookstores, storytelling, and libraries is a conduit in which imagination is absorbed through osmosis.

Using Children's Books in Groups

Both in therapy and in teaching, children's books can be used as jumping-off points to write about deeply buried memories, feelings, creativity, and associations, for example. Both of us, previously unbeknownst to each other, have been using the book, *Harold and the Purple Crayon* (Johnson, 1955/1983) in our academic teaching of expressive arts therapy, on two sides of the world, in two different ways. As you read the following, you might invent a new way to use the book yourself.

In Krystal's class, she invites the students to listen to her read *Harold and the Purple Crayon* aloud. The students sit quietly and listen, this might be the first time they have had a story read to them since they were children or ever. Some might know the story and some may not. After the story is read, the students are asked to turn to a person next to them and form a pair. The pair decides on a role to play; either adult or child. Krystal hands out drawing paper and fat purple crayons to all participants. The "children" are asked to draw on a piece of paper as they tell an adventurous story from their childhood out loud. Each "child" is encouraged to share an adventure similar to Harold's experience. While the "child" is telling their story the "adult" writes the story down on a separate piece of paper. It is important to mention that the "child" is asked to use their non-dominant hand to draw their illustrative picture. This is done to physically remind the students of the concept of control and non-control and to invite more playful yet very challenging drawings. After the drawing and writing is complete the "child" is asked to hold up their drawing while the "adult" reads the story to the whole class. This has become an illustrated children's book. Each pair has a chance to read aloud and share their co-created and illustrated storybook with their classmates without responses. In the next step, the students go back to their pairs and discuss the experience of writing and drawing together. The students may express emotional responses, physical responses, memories, associations, and anything else they feel comfortable sharing. Krystal continues to use this activity with *Harold and the Purple Crayon* year after year as a way of demonstrating the use of children's literature in therapy practice, an integrated arts approach with storytelling, art, and creative writing, as an example of reaching children and adults. As the activity ends, Krystal says aloud, *we are now leaving the role play as "adult" and "child," and we are back to ourselves.* Then, Krystal closes the activity by asking the pairs to thank each other for listening, witnessing, and sharing their stories. One of the questions Krystal asks the pairs to think about is if they felt like they were heard or if their story was understood.

In Tamar's graduate second-year art therapy summer intensives she opens the semester by reading *Harold and the Purple Crayon*, in Hebrew, to get the imagination flowing, and the ability to reconnect to art as accidental, unplanned, and spontaneous, as Harold does. To flow with imagination, to children's stories as problem-solving, and the symbol of home and why it is so important to find it; to see and hear the responses before a six-hour day focused on imagination, creativity, and play. Associative words are written down by the students once the story time ends, they look at them, create a quick line drawing, and then come back to the circle. The sharing includes emotions, memories, and questions about the book, their writing, and their creative process. This opening ritual, which has been going strong for 13 years, is a wonderful way to slowly move into deep days of artmaking and self-reflection.

Shout Out to Children's Books

Shout out to the title of the following children's books. If you resonate and remember any of the books we mention, please feel free to shout their names as you read them, as well as other books that we have not included. We'd like to say a few words about each of these books and their importance to us. Our description of each of the following books is personal, this is our version of seeing the books, and you may have a different interpretation or memory.

- *Ferdinand the Bull* (Leaf, 1936): This book refers to how not fitting in can work to your benefit in the end; remembering one's authentic identity and not losing sight of who you are. Supportive relationships and connections are important; it takes a village to raise an atypical bull. Mistakes can cause major misunderstandings, or don't ever sit on a bee. Ouch!
- *The Little Prince* (Saint-Exupery, 1943): Many stories inside of one long journey; each one is a gem in a treasure chest that one never gets tired of opening. For example, the opening of the first chapter beautifully exemplifies how adults use their brains more than their imaginations, according to children.
- *Frederick the Mouse* (Lionni, 1967): While all of the mice are collecting what they need to survive the winter, Frederick decides that imagination is necessary for survival during winter hibernation. Though his fellow mice don't exactly understand what it is that he is collecting, in the end, they are happy to use his findings.

- *Charlotte's Web* (White & Williams, 1952): On a farm, in a barn, a talented and warm-hearted female spider becomes best friends with a baby piglet. She then, through writing messages in her web, saves him as he grows and becomes a large attractive pig. Also, a story about love and loss.
- *Strega Nona* (dePaola, 1975): A witch whose magical specialty is cooking pasta takes on a helper who mistakenly, though probably as a good deed, blunders, and only the witch has the power to undo this slip-up. Make sure you are hungry before reading this book.
- *The Carrot Seed* (Krauss, 1945): An extremely short and simple children's book that teaches about patience, caring, growth, and believing in yourself; especially if adults don't believe in you.
- *Caps for Sale* (Slobodkina, 1940): A tired hat peddler takes a nap under a tree between walking with hats on his head. He wakes up realizing that the hats are no longer on his head which leads to an adventure to get them back. The story shows perseverance, careful observation of behaviors, and knowing how to use them to one's advantage, and *monkey see monkey do*.
- *Stone Soup* (Brown, 1947): Three hungry and weary soldiers wander to a village seeking food and shelter. After the villagers claim they have no food, the soldiers teach them how to make soup from three large smooth stones, and just a few more ingredients that the villagers eagerly decide to add in. One can make something from anything.
- *Harriet the Spy* (Fitzhugh, 1964): Harriet is a pre-teen who keeps a journal about all the people in her life. This journal is very detailed and personal. The journal is found, which is horrifying to her, and even her beloved babysitter could not calm her down. She eats only one kind of sandwich always. Just one of the quirks we discover about her and her classmates in this coming-of-age classic.
- *There's No Such Thing as a Dragon* (Kent, 1975): A child tries to convince his mother that he has seen a dragon. She refuses to believe this until she has no choice. This book reminds us to listen to children, even if we think they are imagining, or *making up stories*.
- *Something Else* (Cave, 1998): A book that shows children including those who are different from them physically, emotionally, racially, and/or culturally is, in the end, not a deficit, but something you gain from.
- *Madeline* (Bemelmans, 1939): A young girl who lives with other young girls falls ill and is well taken care of. This story has many layers; trust, seeing shapes and beings in shadows, listening, believing, and community.
- *Horton Hatches the Egg* (Seuss, 1940): A gullible, kind, and innocent elephant is "asked" to sit on an egg in a nest high up in a tree. The story takes you on a wild journey that ends up with a happy ending for Horton and the hatchling; fabulously surrealistic. One might learn about self-care, selfishness, bullying, selflessness, fairness and unfairness, and magical endings.
- *Mike Mulligan and his Steam Shovel* (Burton, 1939): A man and his beloved steam shovel do a job they were told could not be done, and find themselves

in a predicament that a child's suggestion solves. This book can show creative solutions, sticking with one's belief in oneself and a work partner, and change coming out of complexities.

- *The Snowy Day* (Keats, 1962): A young boy enjoys a snow day in his snow-covered city, making footprints and snow angels, and whacking snow from the snow-packed trees, ultimately carrying a snowball in his coat pocket to show his mom. This book might be the first children's book to portray a black child as the focus of a wonderful story.

While we realize that many of these books are from a certain generation and are not very diverse in the backgrounds of their authorship, the stories were what were read to us as children and have been carried with us through today.

Re-Discovering our Favorite Childhood Authors in Adulthood: Who Knew?

Maurice Sendak used his children's stories as a way to depict his childhood memories and experiences. According to an article in *Kveller*, the name of the book, *Where the Wild Things Are* (1963) was based on the Yiddish term *vilde chaya*, which Sendak was called by his refugee relatives when he was naughty and sent to bed without dinner (Sorensen, 2022). Sendak took inspiration from his family when he rendered the "things" (monsters) in the story. Sendak referred to his characters as "things." Sendak grew up "in the shadow of the holocaust [and that his parents]... had problems emotionally and mentally" (Sorensen, 2022, para 6).

Kveller reported that Sendak felt lonely and misunderstood as a child. Like many children do, he used stories to escape this harsh reality. Feeling like an outsider explains why Sendak reportedly lived as a recluse into adulthood (Sorensen, 2022). Sendak's books and the shadows and joys they contain, metaphorically and through their illustrations, are exactly why we believe so strongly in using his books and other authors' books in both academic and clinical settings.

One of Krystal's favorite childhood poets was the quirky yet reverent Shel Silverstein. Did you know that Silverstein not only wrote and illustrated his own poems, but he was also a brilliant guitarist and songwriter? According to Biography.com (2023), Silverstein won a Grammy award in 1970 for his song, "A Boy Named Sue" which he wrote for the famous musician Johnny Cash. He was also nominated for both the Academy Award and Golden Globe for his song "I'm Checkin' Out" which was featured in the 1990 film *Postcards from the Edge* (Calley & Fisher, 1990).

Judy Blume has authored many books, infamously including *Are You There God? It's Me Margaret* (1970). To date, that book has celebrated 50 years in print and was recently made into a film. Blume has found a way to stay connected to books at an older age and in a new way. She opened a bookstore in Key West,

Florida. According to an interview with *The Associated Press*, "the author has sold millions of books and still gets approached by adults who teary-eyed, thank her for such meaningful childhood profound experiences" (Italie, 2023, para 1). Tamar read and reread *Are You There God? It's Me Margaret*, over and over when she was a young teenager; and would also probably approach Judy Blume with enormous gratitude and tears were she to see her in person.

Exploring Childhood Autobiographical Writing

Childhood autobiographical memories run the spectrum from the nicest to the most horrifying. Linda Berman's (1993) book aptly titled, *Beyond the Smile: The Therapeutic Use of the Photograph*, refers to the smiles one is asked to produce automatically for photos. When everyone is smiling in the photo, it doesn't mean that they are smiling on the inside. Childhood memories are often not what you see in a family album, they can be masqueraded.

The benefits of recalling our childhoods for people who had happy childhoods or less happy childhoods or both are the raw materials that we work with when we teach and when we use autobiographical writing with our clients and participants. The themes that arise, once written, are then more accessible because they are now outside. The memories have moved from being hidden to being exposed. People have a deep need to tell their stories; this is the beginning of their autobiographical story.

Sometimes delving into childhood memories can bring up traumatic and painful experiences, but shining a light on our childhood and writing about them in detail can give us, perhaps, new ways of seeing behaviors, habits, and how one imagines things, and how they are seen now. Sometimes childhood memories are not about books, they are about foods or smells, sensory-based. People are often shocked by what they can recall by thinking of a smell from their childhood, or a taste, or texture. This connects to family photos, where one's visual memories from photographs may be accompanied by the other senses. Revisiting childhood memories through our senses can help us to make sense of our adult lives. This includes a deeper a listening to ourselves.

In Silverstein's poem, "The Voice," published in *A Light in The Attic* (Silverstein, 1981, p. 137), the conscience speaks to the reader offering some sage wisdom. For Krystal, Silverstein's, "The Voice," and many of his other writings directly spoke to and impacted her in that she resonated with the silliness and a different way of looking at things. His poems were affirming by allowing Krystal to feel seen and heard. What other people may have referred to as quirkiness in these poems and in describing Krystal as a child, and still as an adult, were actually a language and a way of thinking that felt like home to Krystal, and still do.

Tamar, who was referred to as Tammy in America as a young child, discovered that Harriet in *Harriet the Spy* (Fitzhugh, 1964) ate only tomato and mayo sandwiches every single day at school. This was a joyous revelation for Tammy who ate only lettuce and mayo sandwiches at school every day from kindergarten through sixth grade. When Tammy read this, it made her feel like Harriet was her friend and that someone else was like her.

Our childhood stories are small illustrations of how children's books were able to get us through times in our childhood when we weren't always feeling part of what was going on or feeling different than others. Children's books can serve many purposes for young readers of different ages, and you might have your own example of a children's book that had and may still have meaningful messages that are written on your heart.

Connecting to Childhood Through Writing

When people write about their childhood, interestingly, some can write about very early ages, and some cannot. For example, we both have very early memories of when our siblings were born. This includes for instance where we were when we were waiting for our newborn siblings to come home. Tamar remembers picking up her newborn brother and mother from the hospital, with her father and a new blanket they just bought. Krystal even remembers in detail her mother taking her to an ultrasound appointment. In many different languages of psychotherapy and expressive arts therapy, there is a lot of attention paid to childhood. Part of the attention is based on the origins of psychodynamic theories, which suggest that parents inform much of child development. Now in addition and sometimes in opposition to these theories, much attention has been given to ancestral memories, traumas, histories, and collective experiences. In expressive arts therapy from the start, we were trained to look at ancient forms of transformation, reaching memories, shamanism, and other rituals that came from many, many different cultures, before psychotherapy and psychoanalysis ever existed. Therefore, childhood has an important place in expressive arts therapy; however, it is not the only focus of understanding our clients, patients, participants, or students. The arts are as multileveled as human souls; therefore, we are able through the arts to work with many seasons of life simultaneously. For this reason, we give people warm-up writing prompts to reconnect with the earliest memories they may have forgotten. One way of doing this is by asking the participants to write a list of associative childhood memories:

- The first time you felt rain or snow or jumped in a puddle.
- The first time you saw a body of water.
- The first time you tasted a food you loved and the first time you tasted a food that you hated.
- The first time you smelled something nice.
- If you have a sibling, do you remember when your sibling was first brought home?
- The first time you experienced death or loss.

- Learning how to ride a bike or tie your shoes.
- Your first sleepover, either at someone else's house or when you invited someone over.
- Your first memory of a family or group celebration.
- The first time you wrote something, perhaps your name.
- The first time you lost a tooth.

Once completed, these associative memories can be used for other more developed writing exercises. In the interim, the memories are kept in journals.

Sensing, Scents, and Nonsense

The senses: taste, sight, touch, smell, and hearing, are all part of how writing is offered to the students we teach. It has come to our attention that many people are less aware of certain senses and that writing about them or to them or from them reconnects to these senses in a way that brings up meaningful memories.

The sensations can be labeled in words, which clarifies and amplifies people's abilities to connect to their bodies. It can be dramatic and cathartic to write down or to name the sensations that arise within the body once they are recognized. The process of identifying felt sense is not something that happens quickly, it can be a long-term process and should not be rushed. Both authors come from homes that invited and allowed playfulness with words from as far back as we can remember. Now we welcome that playfulness into our classes and workshops. Adults often forget the play of words, and we often need to remind adults of the childhood words they may have made up or stopped using. As adults, we are slowly trained to transform childhood words into more polite, politically correct, and diplomatic words. The words are referred to as nonsense words by adults and are words that were not nonsensical at all when that person was younger; because of that we, on the other hand, see this as a very no-nonsense topic.

Silly Sounds and Silly Words

In the same way that adults seem challenged by nonsense, they also at times seem challenged by what they call silly words or being silly. We try to incorporate nonsense and silly writing in all of our courses, this includes glossolalia, the practice of using playful sounds in speech or making up new language symbols, or movements (Link & Tomaschek, 2023); including words you make up and define in your own way, words you purposely spell in a new way, words that your autocorrect invents that you feel like keeping, words that people around you make up that you feel like keeping and using, words that either you as a child made up or that children around you make up and are often brilliant. For instance, as Krystal noted in her book, at the age of five, following a discussion they had about music and vibration, her son invented a wonderful new word, *vital-bration*, which he defined as, "that vibration is vital to all existence, to human life, and the universe" (Demaine, 2022, p. 29). His imagination allowed him to invent a new word. Many people did not grow up in homes or experience educational settings where imagination was lauded or fertilized like it was in our own homes, and we realize that we are exceptionally blessed and privileged; we love passing along these blessings to our participants and students.

In Tamar's home, she too was brought up with freedom of expression and imagination. She even had three imaginary friends growing up. Her family took it as seriously as she did and allowed Tammy to set three additional places at the dinner table each night and three additional chairs for her imaginary friends to sit in. Tammy (as she was called when she was little) would serve her friends their food, a special invisible and imaginary food that she prepared for them, in their own places. The food was a delicacy. Tammy's family took this very seriously. The name of the special food was *pepolish*. When inviting adults to write in connection to their childhoods they might have memories connected to imaginary foods: the sense of taste; to *vital-brations*: auditory and tactile; and looking at childhood photographs: visual sensations. All of these senses can be explored through silliness as we did when we were children.

Writing Invitation

1 **Name Acrostic**
   An acrostic invites you to create a word or phrase with each letter in your name. Begin by writing your name vertically on a piece of paper and then add a phrase or word starting with each letter.

   Here is an example of **KRYSTAL**'s name as an acrostic:
   Kool-aid man is
   Really cool and
   Yes, I am glad to know about him, however,
   Sometimes I prefer
   To drink things without sugar, so I am
   Asking for some water with
   Lemon

2 **What Is the Meaning of My Name?**
   Do some research about your given birth name, and see what you find; also, do the same if your name has been changed by you or others, by choice or not, and write about how this all feels. We walk around the world with invisible nametags, what do they say? What do they carry? Write all of the names you have ever been called, both by yourself and others, and give a detailed description of each of those people who carry that name: How old

are they? What is their favorite food? What are they wearing? Where do they live? What do they dream to be in the future? Then look at the sentences or short stories you have written and notice what these different versions of you have or do not have in common. Rewrite it as a short story and if you choose to, illustrate it with photographs from different times in your life in which you used these names.

3 New and Made-Up Words

Have you been told stories about words that you made up in your child-hood? Do you have someone to ask if you made up words when you were little? Do you remember words that you have made up in your childhood or adulthood? If not, we invite you to make up or write down these words now. Look at objects and think of new words for them. No one is look-ing over your shoulder, so don't worry. Your word might be better than the one that was given to the object. Allow your silliness to speak. Allow your imagination to express itself and to break rules about what things are called. Dare to tell others your new words and see if they stick. <u>This</u> is how slang begins!!

4 Your Children or the Child in You

In his book *The Prophet*, Khalil Gibran (1923) wrote, "Your children are not your children. They are the sons and daughters of Life's longing for itself. They come through you but not from you, and though they are with you yet they belong not to you." (Gibran, 1923, p. 21).

Is there a sentence, word, or emotion that you feel called upon to research more deeply through writing? If so, sit down, and write the sentence, thought, word, feeling, association, and memory, on the top of the page. Begin writing without using your mind, if possible. Write from your hand connected to your heart and soul. Are you writing as someone's child, parent, or other human, are you on a completely different path than where you imagined this would take you? Stay with the flow. There are many messages that this excerpt can hold, explore them all.

5 Childhood Photo

Find a family album, an actual book album or online. This search might be the beginning of the exercise in itself, the photos might not be where you are and you might have to ask others, family, friends, etc. Look through the photos, and find one of yourself, at any age. Try to remember how it felt to have this photo taken. Who took the photo? Where were you? Who was not in the frame? If there were people with you, what do you remember about your relationships with them? Write freely about this in as much detail as possible. If there is anything you feel you want to change about the photo, you may do it through Photoshop or any other online photo editing software, or you may print out the picture, make a collage, and give it a title.

Resources

Books

Frindle is a wonderful children's book series where the main character has imaginary friends. It is written by Andrew Clements and published in 1996 by
Simon and Schuster Children's Publishing Edition. You can also learn more about the series on the author's website: https://www.andrewclements.com/books/frindle.

Videos

In this 2009 video *Under Squam Rock*, pioneering expressive arts therapist, Shaun McNiff, takes a moment to discuss his surroundings and how they affect him and his art. It was uploaded on February 13, 2009, to McNiff's YouTube channel. You can find it at this link: https://www.youtube.com/watch?v=feGmBrLI5J4.

On the Hearts and Heroes Read Alouds YouTube channel, you can find a book reading of *Harold and the Purple Crayon* by Crocket Johnson. It was uploaded on April 26, 2018 and here is a link: https://www.youtube.com/watch?v=yl94zwz8cKU.
On the Snug as a Bug YouTube channel, you will find a book reading of *Horton Hatches the Egg* by Dr. Seuss. It was uploaded on April 26, 2017 and here is a link: https://www.youtube.com/watch?v=IUgunDvBl90.

Newsletters

In this January 21, 2016, article, "The Eternal Child Inside, Maurice Sendak on Storytelling and Creativity," in *The Marginalian*, Maria Popova describes how Sendak reflected on his childhood to write some of his stories. You can read it here: https://www.themarginalian.org/2016/01/21/maurice-sendak-studs-terkel/

Places

If you are in New York City, check out Bemelmans Bar, a fabulous restaurant painted with illustrations from the children's book *Madeline.* Here is a link to their website: https://www.rosewoodhotels.com/en/the-carlyle-new-york/dining/bemelmans-bar. You can also read a December 10, 2010, review of the bar in *Condé Nast Traveler* by Alex Van Buren at: https://www.cntraveler.com/bars/new-york/bemelmans-bar.
In England, you can visit the Roald Dahl Museum in Great Missenden. Learn more on their website: https://www.roalddahl.com/museum/.
In west central Massachusetts, specifically in Springfield, you can visit the Dr. Suess Museum. Learn more on their website: https://springfieldmuseums.org/seussinspringfield/.

Also in west central Massachusetts, specifically in Amherst, you will find the Eric Carle Museum. Learn more at their website: https://www.carlemuseum.org/.

To learn more about Books and Books @ The Studios of Key West, a bookshop co-founded by the author, Judy Blume, check out their website: https://booksandbookskw.com/.

Famous and Weird Libraries

Fodor's Travel highlights 11 special and stunning libraries around the world, that any book lover would enjoy visiting. Learn more on their January 14, 2023, online article, "Stroll Through the Most Unique Libraries in the World" by Ulrike Lemmin-Woofrey at: https://www.fodors.com/news/photos/the-most-unique-libraries-in-the-world.

Similarly, *Architectural Digest* shares gorgeous libraries that we hope you will feel inspired to visit in this August 3, 2023, article from Katherine McLaughlin, "The 13 Most Beautiful Libraries in the World" at: https://www.architecturaldigest.com/gallery/most-beautiful-libraries-in-the-world

References

Bemelmans, L. (1939). *Madeline.* Simon and Schuster.

Berman, L. (1993). *Beyond the smile: The therapeutic use of the photograph.* Routledge.

Biography.com (2023, August 11). *Shel Silverstein.* https://www.biography.com/authors-writers/shel-silverstein

Blume, J. (1970). *Are you there God? It's me, Margaret.* Simon and Schuster.

Brown, M. (1947). *Stone soup.* Aladdin.

Burton, V.L. (1939). *Mike Mulligan and his Steam Shovel.* Puffin Books.

Calley, J. (Producer), & Fisher, C. (Writer). (1990). *Postcards from the edge* [Film]. Columbia Pictures.

Cave, K. (1998). *Something else.* Mondo Pub.

Demaine, K. (2022). *The roots and rhythm of the heart: Our musical connection to identity, sprit, and lineage.* Lightning Source.

dePaola, T. (1975). *Strega Nona.* Prentice-Hall Inc.

de Saint-Exupéry, A. (1943) *The little prince.* Harcourt Brace & Co.

Dickinson, (2018/2022). The Japanese call this practice tsundoki, and it may provide lasting benefits. *Big Think.* https://bigthink.com/neuropsych/do-i-own-too-many-books/

Etymonline (n.d.). Curiosity (n.). In *Online Etymology Dictionary*. Retrieved December 18, 2023, from https://www.etymonline.com/search?q=curiosity

Fitzhugh, L. (1964). *Harriet the spy.* Harper & Row.

Gibran, K. (1923). On children. In *The Prophet* (pp. 21–22). Knopf.

Italie, H. (2023, April 21). Judy Blume on top of the world (and her Key West bookstore). *The Associated Press.* https://apnews.com/article/judy-blume-profile-65c6a568b562c013bd3306c14cc35417

Johnson, C. (1955/1983). *Harold and the purple crayon.* HarperCollins.

Keats, E.J. (1962). *The snowy day.* Viking Press.

Kent, J. (1975). *There's no such thing as a dragon.* Golden Press.

Krauss, R. (1945). *The carrot seed*. Harper & Brothers.

Landy, R. (1993). The child, the dreamer, the artist, the fool: Understanding the meaning of expressive therapy. *The Arts in Psychotherapy, 20*(5), 359–370.

Leaf, M. (1936). *Ferdinand the bull*. Viking Books for Young Readers.

Lederer, R. (1991). *The miracle of language*. Pocket Books.

Link, S., & Tomaschek, F. (2023). Predictability associated with reduction in phonetic signals without semantics - The case of glossolalia. *Language and Speech*. https://journals.sagepub.com/doi/10.1177/00238309231163170

Lionni, L. (1967). *Frederick the mouse*. Pantheon.

McNiff, S. (2003). *Creating with others: The practice of imagination in life, art, and the workplace*. Shambhala.

Petelin, R. (2022). *How writing works: A field guide to effective writing* (2nd ed.). Routledge.

Seuss, T. (1940). *Horton hatches the egg*. Random House.

Sheldon-Dean, H. (2023. October 27). Why is it important to read to your child? *Child Mind Institute*. https://childmind.org/article/why-is-it-important-to-read-to-your-child/

Silverstein, S. (1981). *A light in the attic*. HarperCollins.

Slobodkina, E. (1940). *Caps for sale*. W. R. Scott.

Sorensen, K. (2022, February 15). *Where the Wild Things Are* is a love letter to Jewish children. *Kveller*. https://www.kveller.com/where-the-wild-things-are-is-a-love-letter-to-jewish-children/

White, E. B., & Williams, G. (1952). *Charlotte's web*. Harper & Brothers.

Chapter 7

A Body of Writing
Writing From, On, and With the Body

Krystal Leah Demaine and Tamar Reva Einstein

Welcome Mat: This chapter will explore the words and images that we hold in and on the body. An exploration of what the authors hold and place in their symbolic and literal meanings will be discussed. Some of the topics will include tattoos, body sounds, body-originated writing, and stories that the body tells. As Lee and Miller-Kristberg poignantly wrote, "...we all have at least one book hiding in the body" (1994, p. xiv).

Writing From the Tip of Your Toes to the Top of Your Head

The word "soma" comes from the ancient Greek word meaning *body*. Somatic or body-oriented writing is a cornerstone of expressive arts therapy; inviting personal and expressive narrative from the body. When one embodies something; physical awareness and a sense of being alive in one's own skin are awoken. Such embodiment can be cultivated and activated through breathing, stretching, drumming, hand clapping, dancing with scarves, tapping, twirling, wiggling, rolling, bouncing, or guided imagery. In expressive arts therapy, which is a body-connected practice, one can add painting, sculpting, mark-making, singing, and playing instruments to amplify one's connection to the body; like that first yawn of the morning when you open your eyes. Anais Nin, writes about the sensual; the utter enjoyment of having a body, a metaphor of a musical crescendo, "The body is an instrument which only gives off music when it is used as a body. Always an orchestra, and just as music traverses walls, so sensuality traverses the body and reaches up to ecstasy" (Nin, 1970, p. 36). From a different viewpoint, based on Eastern thought, B. K. S. Iyengar also relates to music and the body, "Yoga is like music: the rhythm of the body, the melody of the min, and the harmony of the soul create the symphony of the life" (Iyengar et al., 2006, pp. xx–xxi).

We all have a body. Bodies come in different shapes, sizes, colors, challenges, abilities, and many other details with which we describe and in which we have lived since we were born. We have different relationships with our bodies for many reasons. The body's largest organ, the skin, can be considered the container

DOI: 10.4324/9781003391876-8

of this ingenious creation that holds information that can, at times, be hidden. Metaphorically speaking, this body information can be hidden in secret rooms like the four chambers of our hearts; or visible on our skin, represented with birthmarks, scars, wrinkles, or body hair. When we connect writing to the body, because of the intimacy that working with the body brings, we create ways in which to warm up both the body through relaxation exercises, stretching, or engagement of the senses. Warming up the body, in our opinion, must be done with fragility and softness, in the same way that our bodies can sometimes feel fragile and soft. Each of us warms up the body and atmosphere in many ways at different times.

In Krystal's class, she brings her students to a black box theater at the college where she teaches in Beverly, Massachusetts. A black box theater is a theatrical space that is completely black and windowless. In the theater, the students are invited to lie on a yoga mat. Krystal has chosen this room for her work with the body because there are no incoming distractions or disruptions; one can focus solely on oneself. This level of focus and solitude may feel foreign to people and can therefore bring up strong emotions. Some people find the black box theater very calming and others very disturbing. Tamar thinks this room could remind people of a womb, a cocoon, or those indoor personal forts we built when we were children with sheets over tables. It also could remind people of a dark room where photographs are developed. Indeed, in a way, each of Krystal's students is about to develop themselves in the dark.

Krystal prepares the students by asking them to dress warmly and to bring a blanket on the day they go to the black box. She wants the students to feel cozy, encompassed by warmth, and comfortable while lying on a mat, which each student rolls out on a self-chosen spot in the room. Krystal explains the process of *yoga nidra*, or sleep yoga, an ancient form of yoga dating back to around 1000 BC (Pandi-Perumal et al., 2022); a method of relaxing and bringing the body and mind to a place in between falling asleep and staying awake; like the moment before you fall asleep at night. She reads aloud *Yoga Nidra 1*, a script from *Yoga Nidra*, as originally written by Swami Satyananda Saraswati (1976/2009), who defines yoga nidra as, "sleep with a trace of awareness" (p. 17). She asks the students to adjust their clothing and blankets and to lay comfortably because, according to the ancient writings, they will not be moving for the duration of the reading. The yoga nidra script focuses on tuning into the somatosensory system by visualizing micro-locations on both the right and left hemispheres of the body, breathing from different spaces within the body, and imagining colorful scenes. Saraswati suggests that 30 minutes of yoga nidra equals 2.5 hours of restful body relaxation.

When the yoga nidra practice ends, Krystal very slowly invites her students, once they are "awake," to write down in their journal all of the words, images, and sensations they recall from the experience. Their words may turn into reflective phrases or paragraphs. Once everyone has taken the time to write, they are asked to share their thoughts with a partner, noticing common themes or similarities, emotions, sensations, thoughts, or visualizations.

Buddhist meditation teacher and author, Tara Brach (2020), reminds her students and listeners to name the sensations, thoughts, emotions, or feelings that are felt in their bodies. There is an importance Brach suggests in first recognizing the sensation and then giving a name to it, and allowing it to be there. She tells her students to whisper the names of the words and welcome them in. Brach says, "Naming sensations helps us recognize what is happening inside of the body" (p. 43). Krystal continues the ritual of exposing her students to yoga nidra specifically in a space that is very different from most places where they spend their days, and at a pace which they are quite unfamiliar with. This slowing down and deep paying attention is then reflected upon in a short written piece that Krystal receives at the end of the day. Many students report they had never experienced anything like the yoga nidra class before and that it left a deep impression on their bodies and their brains. In closing this body, spirit, and soul practice, Krystal reminds the students that when they leave this dark space, the real world awaits them outside; and that one should be aware and careful of this moving from the slower inner world to the fast outer world.

On a hot summer Tel Aviv day during a three-day summer intensive, Tamar begins the first day, which is about imagination and creativity, with balloons. This is quite surprising to the second-year ultra-orthodox Jewish women students. The students, who traditionally cover their heads, have been told ahead of time to arrive in comfortable clothes, meaning skirts that one can move in, and to perhaps put aside the wigs they wear to cover their heads and bring a fabric head covering so that they can move freely, and not be concerned about art materials like paint getting on their wigs, and still stay modest. Tamar turns off the lights and invites the women to take off their shoes. A gentle and slow body warm-up is done from the tip of the head to the bottom of the feet as a way to connect to their bodies. And then the fun starts.

Tamar goes behind the desk, takes out a bag of balloons, passes it around, and asks the women to choose a color that speaks to them, blow up the balloon, and tie it with a knot. Once each woman, including Tamar, has chosen a color that she wants, Tamar invites them to begin playing with the balloon by gently passing the balloon between their hands while they stay in one place and slowly widening the space between their hands, so gradually the movement becomes bigger and bigger. At this point, usually, the laughter begins. Most of these women have not played with a balloon in a very long time. They are then directed to start moving around the room as they play with their balloon. If they bump into someone that is OK. Tamar tells them to keep moving and that no one is allowed to let their balloon drop to the floor; the balloon must stay aloft in the air. The laughter becomes stronger.

The next step is that Tamar invites the ladies to begin using other parts of their bodies to keep the balloons in the air: shoulders, elbows, heads, back of their body, feet, ankles, hips, nose, and derriere. They use parts of their body to keep their balloon in the air for a few minutes. Then, they are asked to start passing the balloons to each other in no apparent order but remembering that no balloon is allowed to touch the floor. A beautiful colorful chaotic choreography begins with people catching balloons before they hit the floor. The laughter is uncontrollable, and people are sweating. Tamar then says that it is time to freeze with whatever balloon you are holding, even if it is not your original one, to look around the room and observe what it looks like. Then, the women are asked to retrieve their colored balloon from whoever is holding it and to go back to their seat, drink some water, place the balloon down, and write for 10 minutes about the entire experience from beginning to end.

Tamar needs to mention that as the day progresses, they are asked to draw a picture with an oil pastel using the same color as the balloon they chose, then pour gouache paint in the three primary colors: yellow, blue, and red onto a plate. The students then place the balloon in the paint and begin using it to push paint onto enormous pieces of paper that have been hung out the wall. They paint using rolling, pressing, and tapping motions, and adding pressure on the balloon with different parts of their hands and arms. Once the painting is finished, students return to their original seats and are asked to write for another 10 minutes about the experience, the process, and the product. The room is completely transformed, as are their clothes.

When the women sit in the circle to share, there is a lot of discussion about freedom of movement, freedom of expression, and connecting the body to the balloons in many different ways. Students also become very attached to their balloons. Many of the women save it and look at it the next day as the paint has dried on it, they peel the paint off and turn the peeled paint into a collage, yet another transformation. If the balloon pops while the paint is on it, which causes quite a "mess," sometimes the women use the popped balloon in the work that is done the next day.

This series of balloon exercises is something that Tamar has been doing for 14 years in her summer teaching intensives and has noticed how the students become connected to the possibilities and potentials of what their bodies can do and feel in a light-hearted manner. However, what follows sometimes in the writing can connect the women to deeply sad, disturbing, and other feelings. The gift of intermodal expressive arts therapy and writing is that we can research and respect dichotomies and juxtapositions of feelings that arise.

Both Krystal's and Tamar's examples exemplify their intermodal expressive arts therapy roots as they take their students through the body and into other art forms that are very different, yet very similar. Lying flat on the floor quietly to rambunctiously hitting balloons in the air; both are then connected to visual arts and reflective writing. As we mentioned before, all arts begin with the body.

Mapping the Body: Charting the Hidden Safe Passages

In our experience, we have seen body mapping used by different professions to work with participants, clients, and patients on body-related narratives, stories, challenges, medical and mental illness, addictions, food awareness, traumas, aging, and joyous celebrations. When we refer to body mapping, we mean the different ways that the shape of the body can be used as a blank canvas on which personal stories can be told. This can be done by actually tracing around one's own body, allowing someone else to trace the body, or bringing in pre-prepared body stencils and shapes of different sizes.

According to de Vignemont (2017) in the book, *Mind the Body: An Explora-tion of Bodily Self Awareness*, the use of drawing a visual "body map" to under-stand the sensations within the body was first developed by Pierre Bonnier in 1905, who termed the process, "body schema" (p. 84).

People might have self-judgmental thoughts and emotions, painful histories, joyous memories, and sometimes traumas connected to their bodies; there-fore, when inviting participants to create body maps, one should enter these uncharted territories slowly with a compass and with great care. When Tamar co-led groups of adults at a trauma center with a social worker who was a spe-cialist in trauma work, they combined the languages of expressive arts therapy with that of trauma-focused therapies. One of the most meaningful exercises was body mapping. This was done in session seven out of twelve sessions, when the group had created a sense of trust both between themselves and with the facilita-tors. Large pieces of paper were put on the floor and only the facilitators were allowed, after being given permission, to trace the participants' bodies. Because the clients were referred to the trauma center and had undergone lengthy intake sessions with the facilitators, their stories of trauma and post-trauma were known ahead of time. This was not a homogenous group; there were victims of terrorist attacks, rape, car accidents, work accidents, kidnappings, violent domestic situ-ations including divorce, combat stress reaction, and childhood sexual abuse.

Once the body maps were traced, the participants were given 30 minutes to either write words, draw symbols, collage pictures, or place objects on parts of their paper body that had stories to tell. The group reconnected in a circle with body maps on the floor and participants in their chairs; here they shared, wit-nessed, responded, and listened deeply to the stories that were told. Many people chose not to tell their stories that day and asked if they could do it next time. The facilitators completely respected the participant's choices. Those who did not share were asked to tell the facilitators how they felt and to make sure, along with the other participants, to do a closing ritual that contained the emotions that arose during this powerful arts-based experiential therapeutic process. One cannot allow people to walk out of the door of a trauma-based body experiential without there being a very clear closure.

A week later, participants returned to the body maps and were asked to re-share or share for the first time and then write reflectively. They were invited to add or change the body maps to reflect on what they felt that day and to add any new memories, thoughts, or feelings that had arisen over the week. Tamar cannot stress enough how important it is when working with such traumatized participants that the closure of such sessions must be airtight. As Maya Angelou painfully described in, *I Know Why the Caged Bird Sings* (1969/2009) one of the greatest challenges we have is carrying the secrets of body-connected trauma.

In graduate academic settings, Tamar uses very small templates from five to ten inches tall that are very basic shapes and quite gender-free body maps. She hands them out to the students and then shows them a clip from the documentary *Thin* (Greenfield, 2006) in which an art therapist uses body mapping to work with a young woman who is in a live-in facility for people with eating disorders. After viewing the short but disturbing video, the students were asked to draw their own body shape onto the template they were given. It often takes people a long time to begin this exercise. When the students are done, they are asked to write in their reflective journal. A closing discussion ends this class. In their end-of-semester papers, almost all of the students refer to the *Thin* video and the body map they made in class. This, in Tamar's opinion, shows how much there is to be uncovered about one's relationship to their body through the arts in a safe space.

In Krystal's undergraduate therapeutic writing class, students are given a piece of drawing paper a little taller and wider than their own bodies. They are asked to find a partner who they could work with to trace an outline of their body on the paper. The students take turns lying flat on the paper in whatever position they would like to have their bodies traced. They are given time to draw, write, color on, paint, collage, and any other art form they choose to use to illustrate and ornament the life-sized body drawing to illustrate a map of their bodies. These illustrations are focused on the stories that the parts of the body want to tell. The next step of this exercise is for the students to write self-reflectively in their journals while looking at the body maps they have created. Krystal gives the students writing invitations related to different body parts. These might include: What is your hand doing, feeling, holding, sensing, pushing away, and grasping? What color, energy, or sensation is your heart emanating? What words are running through your veins? What have your feet walked through, on, and in, and how does it feel to carry the weight of the whole body throughout the day, and where do you feel that weight? The schema of the body becomes a space in which the exploration of stories carried in the inner organs and the outer protective skin can be exposed and retold in a multi-modal narrative.

Both authors have reached the conclusion after many years of working with body mapping in many different situations, that most people have queries, feelings, and thoughts about their body images.

Writing on the Body

The body is a blank canvas on which stories have been told for thousands of years from tattoos to henna tattoos, to body painting, to covering the skin with mud and other natural substances. Some artists use writing on the body to express and address deep-seated geopolitical and sometimes gender-based inequalities. For example, exiled Iranian artist, Shirin Neshat (1994), exhibited her portrait series titled, "Women of Allah," which integrated body-adorned writing with photography. Within the series, Neshat, an outspoken feminist, chose, in an auto-biographical portrait, to be photographed wearing a black hijab with a poem in handwritten classic calligraphy, in the Farsi language, using black ink across her entire face, titled "Rebellious Silence." The title and image are meant to communicate the power of language on the body.

Face painting is another way to adorn the body with text and mark-making. Tamar uses face painting in both clinical and academic settings. The focus and reason that she uses this particular form of adornment is the immediate transformation that occurs when one's face is painted or written on. Tamar uses many kinds of professional and theatrical body and face paints. As an expressive arts therapy student, she was introduced to these materials and continues to use them.

When she uses this technique in phototherapy classes, she does so in a double-long class. The process begins by handing out tiny mirrors to all of the participants who are asked to look at their faces from different angles: close up, far away, from below, and from the side; when they feel ready, they take photographs of their reflections in the mirror. This takes some time and coordination, as well as a few moments to warm up; especially after spending some time looking at themselves looking in the mirror and paying attention to things that one may not want to focus on in such a close-up way. Tamar discusses how it feels to view ourselves with such intention and intimacy and then take photographs of it.

Tamar then asks the participants to pay attention to how it makes them feel. She invites them to focus specifically on the parts of their faces they like the least. After the photographs are taken, the mirrors are put down and the students are asked to look through all of the photos they have taken and to choose one to write about reflectively for 10 minutes. Tamar then surprises the students by unpacking a bag of many kinds of face paints, including paints in crayon and stick form and paints that are in palettes like watercolors. All of the paints can be applied with fingers, brushes, and sponges.

The students are then invited to open up the mirrors again and find a place on their face that will be the starting point for where they will begin the face painting; this could be a mole, a scar, a dimple, or a wrinkle. Tamar explains the paints are hypoallergenic. Every once in a while, there is someone who refuses to participate in the exercise for many different reasons; that person is invited to do the exercise on their hand, though once they start this, they often end up painting their face. The words most often spoken about by students with respect to this work are: transformation, change, masquerade, and exposure.

Students are asked to take photographs every few moments so that the stages of transformation are chronologically documented on their cameras. After 45 minutes of face painting, most are unrecognizable, and then they begin to take self-portraits in different lighting, with props, fabrics, objects, and other accouterments that can transform them or frame their faces in the photographs in other ways. The initial rebellion to this experiential activity disappears into complete magical enchantment into what they have become. They are given time to look at the self-portraits and write about how it feels to be transformed, who or what have they been transformed into, and what associative thoughts, imaginations, and stories come up.

Almost every year the class asks Tamar to take a group picture of them in their transformed state. This exercise can bring up many different emotions and ideas. The sharing and closure at the end of this class are very meaningful. By the end, many have washed off their face paint while others choose to drive home with the paint still on their faces. This exercise reminds participants what transformation feels like, what gets exposed that is often hidden, and what people sometimes wear on the outside that is usually worn on the inside. The act of removing the face paint is sometimes as, if not more, meaningful than applying the face paint, a process that is also photographed. The students understand why Tamar repeated the word transformation so many times as she reiterates that therapy is a place where people transform.

Some of Tamar's participants report healing aspects of the face painting, including a student who began painting her face every time she started to get a headache and made a video about this for her final project. Every time she got a migraine, she would start painting, beginning from her temples toward her third eye in different colors, over and over, and she found that this helped her get through her migraine.

A not-too-distant cousin to face painting is tattoos, which have historically been placed on the body for healing, reduction of pain, fertility, against the evil eye, and for many other health and spiritual reasons. According to an article in *Smithsonian Magazine*, tattooing and skin marking are cross-cultural and date back thousands of years (Lineberry & Anderson, 2023). There are many kinds of skin marking and some don't use ink at all. There has simply been a need for people to mark their bodies to communicate or in some cases to heal. People nowadays may not be aware of the history of the tradition or where tattoos come from, they were not just done for fashion, there was a reason. Nowadays people get tattoos like a pieces of jewelry or clothing, though there are people who get tattoos to commemorate rites of passages including births and deaths. Centuries ago, only certain people were allowed to give tattoos and the procedure was part of a ritual. Joann Fletcher wrote that tattoos:

> sprung up independently as a permanent way to place protective or therapeutic symbols upon the body, then a means of marking people out into appropriate social, political or religious groups, or simply as a form of self-expression or fashion statement.
>
> (Lineberry & Anderson, 2023, para 27)

Some tattoo studios are reconnecting with the lost ritualistic aspects of tattooing and receiving tattoos. Tamar has a friend who chose such a tattoo experience and was taken through a ceremony involving guided imagery and a healing ceremony before the tattoo was done. This is a far cry from the Western familiar style of walking into a pitch-black tattoo studio, being handed a Xeroxed album of symbols, words, or quotes to choose from, and then being taken into a back room where a tattoo is done. Tamar, for example, has a small tattoo at the nape of her neck that is an ancient Berber symbol of the tree of life that the women in the mountains of Morocco used to have tattooed in the middle of their forehead for protection. Tamar did this tattoo with a group of four women as a ritual.

Tattoos were once, at least in modern Western society, considered cheap, exotic, barbaric, primitive in a bad way, a sign of being part of a gang or a crime group, or simply carried a stigma (Béreiziat-Lang & Ott, 2019). Many religions prohibit tattoos.

Tamar's beloved tattoo artist told her, that in Russia, the artist's father and friends had large portraits of political leaders tattooed on their entire backs so that they would not get beaten up in prison. The belief was that nobody would hit someone who was in political power for fear of retaliation. This shows the power that tattoos have.

As noted by the Memorial Sloan Kettering Cancer Center (2022), tattoos are used to create three-dimensional nipples for women and victims of breast cancer. Also from the medical world, some people choose to have tattoos of their allergies, illnesses, or end-of-life wishes tattooed on their bodies so that first responders can immediately see them (Gilbert & Boag, 2018). Tattoos were not always done by choice. In the Auschwitz concentration camp, Holocaust victims were tattooed on their forearms with identifying numbers. Today, some ancestors of these Jews are choosing to have the numbers tattooed on their forearms as an act of commemoration and of never forgetting the Holocaust (Pavia, 2023).

When one gets a tattoo nowadays, they are given a clear list of instructions for aftercare; for the wound that once scabbed over to become a permanent tattoo. You are told to go and buy a cream that often has a smell of diaper cream and other childhood ointments. This is a strange juxtaposition of skin care and olfactory childhood memories. Tattoos might be a way, in this confusing and complex world, to have an indelible and permanent mark on our body; an inked transitional object when the world seems so topsy turvy like in *Alice in Wonderland* (Carroll, 1865/2021).

Removing and Keeping the Labels We've Been Given: Labels on the Body

When Krystal was an assistant professor at Lesley University, she heard about an art therapy student who designed a project using writing, labels, and performance. Upon planting the seeds for writing this book, Krystal contacted that student to meet and hear more about the project. The former student, Cacky (real name used with permission), told Krystal that in high school she had been bullied, and upon being given an undergraduate college art therapy mid-term assignment to *explore a relationship*, she decided to explore her relationship with names that she had been called throughout her life including positive, negative, and neutral names. She came up with 500 words! She wrote all of the names with black permanent marker on "Hello my name is" white sticker tags. She said, "The writing felt cathartic but there was more to be done" (C. Mellor, personal communication, May 22, 2023). There was a feeling that something was missing in the process; the writing of the names was just the beginning. Interestingly while on vacation with her family in New York City, she visited Times Square around lunchtime, one of the busiest times of the day there, when thousands of people are quickly walking by. She prepared for the possibility of taking the next step that had been missing with the labels, by wearing specific clothing and carrying the labels with her to this tourist attraction. At some point, she chose a spot, on an asphalt sidewalk island in front of the M&M candy store, and with the help of her mother and sister, stuck all of the labels on her body. The sticking of the labels on her body was reminiscent of a rite of passage ritual. She had intentionally worn a nude-colored short-sleeved leotard so that her clothes would not take attention away from the word labels. She stood still there, smiling as cars, bicycles, and perhaps people dressed in Elmo and Mario Brothers costumes, as well as many other tourists passed her by. She was pushed and nudged on this busy sidewalk. She waved hello to witnesses who showed interest by staring, glimpsing, resonating, and showing a spectrum of different reactions while she stood there on her island for the entire afternoon.

After her performance, when Cacky removed the stickers from her body she found out that she was allergic to the glue on her skin, a bodily reaction to the labels being affixed to her body and perhaps a metaphor for carrying these labels inside of her body for many years. She also found it transformative to rip the labels off afterward. Cacky's "label project" led to her own understanding of how the literal and metaphoric labels in her life have impacted her body, and how labels can be removed. The project informed her to pursue a Ph.D. in depth psychology and work as a somatic experiencing practitioner, helping her clients understand their bodies. At this point, Cacky has performed "the label project" 18 times, all over the world including at Harvard University, the Louvre in Paris, London, and Balboa Park in San Diego, California. Cacky has led workshops to help others explore the labels they write on their selves and the power of removing those words.

When Tamar read this piece about Krystal and Cacky's intimate and moving conversation, she resonated strongly with Cacky's feeling that writing labels felt transformative or cathartic but not enough. When Tamar sewed a multi-cultural coat for her arts-based doctoral studies, she had the same response as the coat hung in her living room on a hanger. Once Tamar started to have people wear the coat and feel it on their bodies and tell Tamar how it felt to wear the symbols, the process felt complete, in the same way, that Cacky's process felt complete when she was able to affix and remove labels while being witnessed. These are two examples of wearing and removing stigmas, symbols, labels, and the transformative power of taking control of that process.

Tuning in and Sounding from the Body

Children and infants easily play with sounds while they are learning language. Infants babble, blow "raspberries," and begin to copy sounds and eventually by the age of three to four years develop fluency in their mother tongue. As children grow older, language acquisition develops, and they lose the sense of playfulness in sounds (Brandt, Gebrian, Slevc, 2012). Sounds in words have emotion, fluctuation, and musicality. When we exaggerate and play with our sounds, they can mean different things.

Krystal encourages verbal sound exploration and play with both her students and in clinical settings. In her classroom, Krystal invites students to explore the syllables and sounds within words. With the students sitting or lying on the floor, Krystal uses the word "home" as a metaphor for the self as body, and asks the students to spell it out letter by letter. She then asks the students to sound the letters of the word one at a time, H—O—M—E. Each letter is vocalized slowly and deliberately, emphasizing the nuances of pitch, vibration, tones, melodies, and contours. Beginning with H, she asks the students to practice saying the "H" with short and long sounds, full and shallow sounds, and notice where in which part of the body the sound originates; is it the throat, the chest, or the abdomen, or felt in any other parts of the body, perhaps the head, the feet? After each letter is sounded, the students write the sensations down in their journals. She then asks students to visualize where each part of the word sits in their body. "H" can begin in the throat, and travel to the middle abdomen; leaving the "H," the sound of "O" travels down to the lower abdomen; then, the sound "M" moves to the lips and cheeks; and "E" is silent almost as a quiet requiem resonating in stillness after the symphony of the word is spoken. When words are slowed down and felt like this, they are almost no longer words as we know them in regular writing, reading, or speaking; they become deeply connected to how we say them and what part of the body is saying them. In this exercise, one feels words through and in the body, which is not how we usually use words in daily communication. However, the authors feel it is important to mention that when words are used to harm, such as in name-calling, one feels those words in the body, though the words are often shut tightly or hidden away and only come to the surface during exercises like this. The English language children's rhyme says, "Sticks and stones may break my bones, but names will never hurt me" (Word Histories, n.d.). Though this adage is from the 1800s, people today can be bullied and have names called at them not just in person but also on social media and online. Those words can etch an imprint on one's soul.

After the writing, the students are asked to review their notes, reread their words, underline areas they resonate with, and write reflectively: poem, prose, short story, list, narrative, or dialogue. Students are given 20 minutes to write and then share their work with the class. Emotional topics tend to emerge, the feelings of pleasure, joy, fear, and sometimes confusion.

Photographing and Writing from the Body: From Standing Still to Take a Still, and Moving to Take a Still

In the Phototherapy Institute in Jerusalem, Tamar connects the act of photographing to moving the body and then to writing. Students are asked to spread out in the room with room to move and to have their camera, or phone with a camera, in their hand. It might be worth mentioning here that movement and photography are quite different art forms. One usually stops moving to take a photograph, as opposed to dance and movement where all parts of the body are explored through moving. So, this combination of these two art forms is foreign, fruitful, interesting, and at times quite surprising to the participants. Once the students have found a comfortable place, they are invited to close their eyes and begin placing the camera on different body parts of the body to take photos; hips, foreheads, elbows, back, heart, toes, anywhere! Once they begin playing in this way they get looser and explore more, taking photos from the nose, the backside, and the ears.... The next step is to continue, with eyes closed, to slowly begin moving around the room while taking photos of body parts; if one bumps gently into another a photo is taken of that too. After this experience, the students sit down and look at all their photos and write. Topics emerge from the intensity of not having the use of the eyes, a photographer's best friend, and from allowing the body to lead what is photographed. Insights are shared; the realization of not feeling in control, or opposingly of pure freedom, thoughts about the photos are also shared; there are surprising angles, lights, and shadows. People discuss how it felt to touch one another as they bumped and grazed. The writings are shared with Tamar in their papers at the end of the semester when they are asked to choose one meaningful photo from each class and its accompanying writing.

The body is a conduit to stories, memories, the shadow, the self, the psyche, the four chambers of the heart and what they hold, and meaningful experiences that flow through the veins, the emotions we breathe in and out, or sometimes freeze when we hold our breath; this holds such riveting writing potential. Humans are story-bound, story-rooted, and storytellers; writing these body-related stories seems so natural and a great prescription for a healthy life practice. Gottschell (2012) takes storytelling a step deeper and leads us to understand that as humans, even when asleep, we continue to tell ourselves stories.

Writing Invitations

1 **Body Paths**

Draw or sketch a body shape, it can be from teeny tiny to very large. On a separate piece of paper begin to write the history of your body chronologically, including any moments that feel important, meaningful, surprising, exciting, painful, confusing, frightening, and/or pleasurable. As you write you might begin remembering things long forgotten: one's first menstrual period, reaching puberty, a bee sting, a wonderfully intimate experience, tasting food for the first time, hearing a piece of music or a voice, getting bad news or good news over the phone, breathing in rancid or glorious scents, surgery, scars, concussions, seeing a vista that left an impression, for example. After you write this list, which can be done over some time: hours, days, or weeks, take out the body shape you drew and write the words with their dates on the places of the body that you feel are their right place. Perhaps use different colors. One may add to this body path whenever it feels needed. Write down how it feels to get to know your body as a chronological container, a path of bodily sensations and memories. Another stage of this might be to connect the events with thin lines and arrows, creating a path. Then write a story, poem, essay, or short story, about "my body's path in life."

2 **Sounding from the Body**

Vocalizing sounds that originate from sensations or emotional places in the body can be a powerful practice for resilience, expression of pent-up energy, and salve for the nervous system. Think of all of the sounds you vocalize innately as a way to self-soothe: a yawn, a sigh, a moan, a groan, a deep exhale or inhale, perhaps paired with a hum, buzz, or hiss, or sometimes even a scream or a cry. Have you ever noticed the quality of these sounds, the depth of breath, the richness in the timbre? Have you ever noticed where these sounds originate from in your body: your legs, abdomen, belly shoulder, throat nose, or perhaps you are not sure? Take a moment to recount and write times when you used audible sounds in your body. Then beginning with the nose, take a few rounds of inhales and exhales noticing the quality of sounds in the nose breath. In your journal, write all of the sounds from your breath, the quality of the sound: airy, full, deep, shallow, blocked. Can you write the word for the sound nose breath: *shhhh, blahh, frrfff,* or something different? Now take the air to the throat, breathe from the throat with the mouth closed; notice the quality of sound, and write down the word that it sounds like. Go to the chest, do the same kind of breathing for a few cycles, and write. Then go to the abdomen and do the same. At this point, do you begin to vocalize with those air sounds, does your mouth open, do your eyes widen, does the shape of your hands, or posture shift? Notice all of the things that happen when you make sounds from different parts of your body, write about what you observe, how you feel, and what you think your body may be communicating or feeling as you express these sounds.

If you feel called to do so, draw an illustration of your body sounds: the spine yelling, the wrists shouting, or the finger crying.

3 **Positive Body Affirmations**

Cut out small shapes of paper: rectangles, squares, hearts, stars, circles, or small body shapes, any shape that speaks to you; large enough to write on, but not too large. On a different piece of paper write down some affirmations. For example: I am blessed, I will follow my intuitions, I am a changing and evolving human, I will take good care of myself, I will practice more self-care, I deserve pauses, I am not perfect and I am beautiful, I am doing my best, life is full of surprises and I will try hard to accept them, I deserve therapy and support, I can ask for help and still be strong, trees have seasons and so do I, that is fine, it is not my fault that I am anxious or depressed, I can say no, and any other self-affirming phrases you make up. After this writing, begin to write the phrases, sentences, or paragraphs on the shapes you cut out. Watch the pile grow, feel what that is like. Keep these and new ones you might add periodically in a container that feels like the right fit: a woven basket, a box, a glass jar.... Does it want to be covered or open? Is this placed in a private or public shared space? Each day reach your hand in and take one out. Read what it says, if you have time meditate on it, perhaps write something, paint something, photograph something, or collage something that resonates with the words. Try this as a daily practice and see how it feels, and what it brings into your day. Maybe end the day similarly.

4 **Writing from the Skin**

The skin covers us, protects us, and is our largest organ. It has pores, it absorbs, it sweats, and it is both fragile and resilient. It has hair and more protection. It is a beautiful rich spectrum of colors and textures. In this writing invitation, imagine your skin writing. What does it have to say, ask, affirm, scream, whisper.... What does it prefer or dislike? Cold showers, hot showers? Hair or hair removal? Get into details. What does your scar want to tell, what do your eyebrows have to say, what stories do your armpits carry, when have your forearms wanted to tell a story, what does the skin on your back remember about a sunburn, are your wrinkles holding memories, and perhaps hidden skin holds tales untold. Write from the skin. Allow the skin to become expressive, and listen to what it has to tell you. If you want to take this a step further, you can actually write the important words, with special hypoallergenic body paints, on those places, giving the skin back some response writing. Take photos. Write about them.

Chapter Resources

Books

A wonderful book about the history of tattoos is *Written on the Body: The Tattoo in European and American History*, edited by Jane Caplan and published in 2000 by Princeton University Press. https://press.princeton.edu/books/paperback/9780691057231/written-on-the-body

Websites

Sengi Mossi is a drawing and dance project for children and adults based in Italy. You can learn more about it on their website: https://www.segnimossi.net/en/.

Videos

Watch this video of Lama Majaj, an expressive arts therapist immersing herself in embodied artmaking, found on the IACAET YouTube channel from September 23, 2020: https://www.youtube.com/watch?v=3AwdbMaEFMQ.

Thin is a recorded art therapy example of body mapping and a girl with eating disorders. You can see it on the april1819 YouTube channel where it was uploaded on October 4, 2006. https://youtu.be/cAw9n7_9eW8.

References

Angelou, M. (1969/2009). *I know why the caged bird sings*. Random House.

Béreiziat-Lang, S., & Ott, M.R. (2019). From tattoo to stigma: Writing on body and skin. In R. Wagner, C. Neufeld, & L. Lieb (Eds.), *Writing beyond pen and parchment* (pp. 193–208). De Gruyter. https://www.degruyter.com/document/doi/10.1515/9783110645446-010/html

Brach, T. (2020). *Radical compassion: Learning to love yourself and your world with the practice of RAIN*. Penguin Books.

Brandt, A., Gebrian, M., & Slevc, L. R. (2012, September 11). Music and early language acquisition. *Frontiers of Psychology, 3*. https://www.frontiersin.org/articles/10.3389/fpsyg.2012.00327/full

Carroll, L. (1865/2021). *Alice's adventures in Wonderland*. The Project Gutenberg. https://www.gutenberg.org/cache/epub/11/pg11-images.html

de Vignemont, F. (2017). *Mind the body: An exploration of bodily self-awareness*. Oxford Academic Press.

Gilbert, J., & Boag, J. (2018). Nonstandard advance health care directives in emergency departments: Ethical and legal dilemma or reality: A narrative review. *Advanced Emergency Nursing Journal, 40*(4), 324–327.

Gottschell, J. (2012). *The storytelling animal: How stories make us human*. Houghton Mifflin Harcourt.

Greenfield, L. (2006). *Thin* [Film]. HBO.

Iyengar, B. K. S., Evans, J. J., & Abrams, D. (2006). *Light on life: The yoga journey to wholeness, inner peace, and ultimate freedom*. Harmony/Rodale.

Lee, J., & Miller-Kritsberg, C. (1994). *Writing from the body: For writers, artists, and dreamers who long to free their voice*. St. Martin's Publishing Group.

Lineberry, C., & Anderson, S. (2023, October 18). The worldwide history of tattoos. *Smithsonian Magazine*. https://www.smithsonianmag.com/history/tattoos-worldwide-history-144038580/

Memorial Sloan Kettering Cancer Center (2022, November 2). About your nipple and areola tattoo procedure. https://www.mskcc.org/cancer-care/patient-education/about-your-nipple-and-areola-tattoo-procedure

Neshat, S. (1994). *Women of Allah* [Photograph series]. The Met, New York City. https://www.metmuseum.org/art/collection/search/486834

Nin, A. (1970). *The diary of Anaïs Nin, 1934–1939*. Houghton Mifflin Harcourt.

Pandi-Perumal, S.R., Spence, D.W., Srivatsava, N., Kanchibhotla, D., Kumar, K., Saurabh Sharma, G., Gupta, R., & Batmanabane, G. (2022). The origin and clinical relevance of yoga nidra. *Sleep Vigil, 6*(1), 61–84.

Pavia, J. (2023). In honor of zaide: A Jewish man explains his Holocaust memorial tattoo as part of Ontario study. *CBC*. Retrieved December 15, 2023, from https://www.cbc.ca/news/canada/kitchener-waterloo/in-honour-of-zaide-a-jewish-man-explains-his-holocaust-memorial-tattoo-as-part-of-ontario-study-1.6865788

Saraswati, S.S. (1976/2009). *Yoga Nidra*. Golden Jubilee (Ed.). Yoga Publications Trust.

Word Histories (n.d.). Sticks and stones may break my bones but names will never hurt me. https://wordhistories.net/2022/05/18/sticks-stones-break-bones/

Chapter 8

Writing on the Inside and the Outside

Boxes, Masks, and Other Containers

Krystal Leah Demaine and Tamar Reva Einstein

Welcome Mat: This chapter discusses the inner and outer, what we expose and what we hide. Exploring how finding parts of the self that are unseen or seen will give the reader insight into how making art informs the writing and vice versa. Though a mask is usually conceived to be something that hides ourselves, it might be doing the opposite, a mask might expose parts of ourselves that we would normally never show in public. Similarly, the inside and outside of boxes might take on opposite meanings of what the art maker began creating; the inside of the box may reveal much more than the outside.

Inside and Outside: Outside and Inside

In our experience, we have noticed that people have both an inner self and an outer self that are often not paid attention to. There is a reason for this, and there are proverbs and sayings that relate directly… *I wear my heart on my sleeve*, for example, offering a figure of speech exposing inner feelings completely outward. When this phrase was first spoken in Shakespeare's play *Othello* it was probably referring to medieval jousting in which secret symbols on a knight's protective arm wear proclaimed secret feelings for female spectators of the sport (No Sweat Shakespeare, n.d.). This adage still sticks with us as a wonderful metaphor for hiding and showing hidden feelings through writing and the arts. Writer, Zadie Smith reiterates the concepts of masking and exposing our feelings when she writes, "Every moment happens twice: outside and inside, and they are two different histories" (Smith, 2003, p. 441).

Boxes, masks, and other containers can be created from a variety of different materials. Boxes can be anything from brown cardboard shipping boxes, metal, wood, plastic, both opaque and transparent, cloth, plasticine, clay, empty cassette and CD containers, paper mâché, plaster strips, glass, clay, found objects such as fruit or vegetable baskets from the supermarket, and colanders. They can be tiny or huge. Similarly, masks can be made from many diverse materials, both found and created, including silver tin foil, brown paper, clay, plaster strips, pre-made masks, paper, wood, natural materials, textiles, and paper mâché. Masks can

DOI: 10.4324/9781003391876-9

be worn or not worn which means they can also be made more temporarily; for example, our contributions as illustrated in Susan Ridley's edited book used objects in a non-permanent way, assemblage (Demaine, 2024; Einstein, 2024).

Other containers refer to anything that contains or could contain matter: bowls, candle holders, two hands cupped together, shoes, upside-down hats, musical instruments, bottle and jar caps of different sizes, 35 mm film containers, old medicine bottles, egg crates, paper towel inner rolls, and shipping containers made of cardboard, fabric, plastic, or paper bags, for instance.

The use of boxes, masks, and other containers is a way of delicately circumventing, probing, and unearthing the feelings, thoughts, and emotions that may be buried deep inside a person. Perhaps thoughts that are not even remembered or feelings and sensations that cannot be felt. When paired with writing and other expressive arts, containers often allow participants to explore their inner and outer treasure chests. At times, the exploration becomes an emotional archeological dig. Ancient hidden feelings must be handled with care, excavated slowly, brushed off gently, sifted finely, witnessed, and documented carefully.

Boxes: Boxed in and Writing Outside of the Box

When we work with boxes, we want to think outside of the box. In other words, we invite participants to use boxes to explore their insides and outsides in a new light, exploring beyond the confining space of the box, both metaphorically and literally. The actual material used can in itself symbolize different aspects, memories, or associations related to the explorations. For example, soft, hard, fragile, transparent, open or closed boxes can have a representational symbol for that person's thoughts, feelings, or spiritual situation at the moment. Boxes can range in size from a matchbox to a refrigerator box, the size chosen can also have deep meaning.

It is common to begin expressive arts therapy processes by discussing expectations verbally and sometimes signing mutual therapeutic expectations and containing agreements, including how the works created will be stored, cared for, and kept safely. At times a box is chosen for this personal safe protective space in which all that is created in the sessions will be contained. These spaces can range from pizza boxes to large cardboard cartons, to plastic boxes with covers, or cubbyholes and drawers, that communicate the same message of safekeeping. Once a box is chosen, the client is invited to ornament, decorate, and write their name on the box. The writing of the name is an important ritual, as it allows the person to take ownership and stewardship over what will be inside. This box and what it will contain is theirs and only theirs. The box can be painted, collaged, used as a place on which to write, or any other way of leaving a personal mark. The names might be big or small, repeated in different places, and worked on for more than one session. Boxes can be reminiscent of treasure chests in which our clients keep their sacred art which holds their sacred emotions and stories (Farrell-Kirk, 2001).

Another way of using boxes is as transitional objects, or talismans, good luck symbols, or portable altars. With a group of 40 school psychologists, Tamar brought 40 tiny matchboxes that she had emptied and painted white beforehand. The participants were asked to choose words from a writing experience done earlier that morning about resilience, war, weaknesses, strengths, affirmations, self-forgiveness, burnout, and guilt. Tamar asked them to look at what they had written and choose sentences that made them feel inspired, relieved, contained, authentic, and cared for. They were then given small slips of paper, fortune cookie size, on which to write these sentences or words, and some added new ones. When everyone had a tiny pile of written gems in front of them, Tamar handed out the teeny matchboxes. Then they were asked to write and/or draw on the boxes, to title them, perhaps. Some drew elaborate small scenes, some wrote, and some doodled... Then the participants were asked to share what their notes said aloud, a group ritual that seemed important and meaningful. Some borrowed others' words and added them. Then all the psychologists carefully placed the slips of paper into their boxes and slid them shut. Tamar discussed these as "grownup" transitional objects in this shocking, complex, and confusing time of the autumn of 2023 in the Middle East. There were many smiles, unusual for that time, some participants were truly enamored by what they had made for themselves, self-gifts! The places they thought they would keep these varied: pocketbooks, desk drawers, on shelves in their home or office, and in their car. Tamar and the psychologists discussed how this box use could be translated for use with the diverse populations with whom they do therapy. Boxes can be safe spaces in many ways, but also feel too constrictive to some. All of this can be addressed as part of the writing about the boxes.

Masks

Masks have an outside and an inside; usually, people focus on the outside. When we use mask-making in groups, both academically and otherwise, the inside is given as much attention and importance as the outside. There is a long-standing ritual that spans thousands of years in most of the world in which masks are used for different traditional and transformative celebrations, rites of passage, ceremonies, and play. Some well-known examples of mask-wearing within such traditions include Venetian Carnival masks, Purim, Carnivale in Brazil, New Orleans Mardi Gras, Mexican Day of the Dead, Halloween, Chinese New Year masks, African Festima masks, and there are many more (Zechner, 2016).

Masks invite crossing boundaries, role play, transformation, and continuity of cultural traditions and rituals. Masks invite people to be something or someone else, even if just for one day of the year. Interestingly, many mask-wearing traditions include lots of preparation for just one day of celebration. Transformation is very important to people; it seems to be an intrinsic human need to feel completely transformed and sometimes the opposite of how someone usually feels when wearing a mask. Furthermore, it often allows one to explore other parts of themselves that they may not be able to do when they are not wearing a mask. As Toni Morrison wrote "The ability of writers to imagine what is not the self, to familiarize the strange and mystify the familiar, is the test of their power" (Morrison, 1992, p. 8).

In Tamar's mask-making classes, plaster strip masks are made. Once the plaster masks are completed, students are asked to do free writing that day (Einstein, 2024). Afterward, once the mask is taken home to be continued over the course of a month, and altered, ornamented, decorated, placed, and photographed in different places, the students are asked to write, in playwriting style, a dialogue between the inside and outside of the mask. This conversation, as a play, allows the inner and outer parts of the student to discuss important topics with one another, as the mask has symbolized. The students are invited to have this written dialogue refer to the mask-making process and product. Tamar assigns the dialogue style of writing that is reminiscent of playwrights for a specific reason. Tamar assumes that the students, like herself and many other humans, have an inner self and an outer self; in different theories, this has been referred to as the self, the subconscious, the conscious, the true self, and the false self; the mask is a very concise art-based metaphor that allows exploration of what we expose and what we keep hidden. Because a mask that is made with plaster strips is extremely close to how one looks, the dialogue with the mask becomes very authentic and personal. For example, there have been dialogues between: my anima and animus sides, my deceased mother and myself, my destructive and self-compassionate sides, and my perfect and imperfect self. The seam connecting the inside and outside of the mask, like the places in ourselves that connect our inner and outer parts might be very thin, but contain years of meaningful information that often isn't revealed until we begin the writing process.

Similarly, Krystal uses plaster mask-making with her undergraduate students to explore their inner and outer selves; this is an initiation into the writing. Once students finish making the masks in class, they are asked to take the mask home and bring them back, transformed creatively, one week later. When the students return to the classroom it has been set up ahead of time with tables and chairs in a large circle. The students sit with their masks and journals on the table in front of them. Krystal asks them to sit quietly looking at their masks as they take time to absorb the details and the whole piece as it has returned after being away; this includes a detailed observational list of everything they see: colors, shapes, forms, objects, textures, in a phenomenological way (Betensky, 1995).

Then Krystal asks the students to engage in a process of image dialogue which our mentor Shaun McNiff trained us to use at Lesley University, but Krystal translates the dialogue into written form, rather than spoken out loud.

As McNiff (1992) wrote, "Image dialogues deepen the creative process," which involves speaking with, to, and from the image (p. 109). This is a very personal way of engaging with an image that many people are not used to; it gives the image a persona, the image is honored by allowing it to speak what it wants to say, and the creator of the image is respected and honored by answering the image. Krystal guides the students through the dialoguing with specific invitations: what is the mask's name, where did the mask grow up, what did the mask do over the weekend, how old is the mask, what is the mask's favorite food, what is the mask's message to you? Of course, one needs to use imagination to answer these questions. The students are ripe and ready to write these image dialogues and jump right into it. It is important to note, that both of us do the mask-making class in the last third of the semester when we know the students well and reciprocal trust has been built.

When the different stages of the writing process are complete, a sharing circle begins. Each student, in turn, shares information that has been given to them or they have learned, or received in the mask dialogue. One by one, they introduce the mask to the class. Then the other classmates are invited to write a handwritten letter directly to that particular mask; this is a form of aesthetic feedback and becomes a ritual round in the circle, and directed toward the mask from different vantage points. By the end of the class, each student has received a letter from each of the witnesses who wrote to that mask. After receiving verbal and written attention, the mask and mask maker go home, and the students are left with more to explore, write, make, and perhaps learn about themselves and their masks. The class might have ended, but the process has just begun.

Masks are sometimes made from small found objects, which is how we made ours when invited to make autobiographical masks for a book on therapeutic mask-making in which we each wrote chapters (Ridley, 2024). As it happens, we each followed our artistic instincts and made masks that were non-permanent without using our faces as the template, though still autobiographical. Both masks were assemblages, which means they were created from objects, assembled and placed in different ways on a flat surface, but not permanently attached.

Krystal's mask was made from small objects from her home with which she has a special relationship. The shape of the mask was made of a variety of differently colored and sized glass marbles, some originally belonging to her grandmother. Additional objects placed around the marbles included bits of lavender flowers, two small Buddha statues, two small frog statues, and magnet words: *play, medicine, understand, trust,* and *journey.* A small red glass heart was placed at the neck of the mask which was surrounded by her son's Star of David bracelet.

Tamar's mask started with two large date palm branches, found after a windy sandstorm, which she placed next to a pre-made mask that she had painted copper. She then placed a crystal on the forehead where the third eye might be. Tamar's assemblage was laid out on a fuchsia-colored shawl placed outdoors.

Both of our mask assemblages were photographed and personally reflected through writing in our journals.

Other Containers

We use a variety of different objects and containers to connect people to associations, memories, and emotions as they write. The types of containers that we choose to work with are intentional and not random. We understand one's reaction to the containers we choose will be expansive and unplanned as the creative exploration unfolds. In other words, we have to plan for the unplannable. We think about the potential reactions people might experience and we often try these experiences out ourselves before introducing them to groups. Within the enormous world of containers, some are bottomless, opaque, transparent, open and closable, pierced, amorphous, invisible or imagined, musical, or physical.

In Krystal's undergraduate expressive arts therapy courses where cultivating imagination and play is key, a very physical group example is that of using an extra-large elastic fabric-covered stretch band, that can expand or retract depending on how much body weight is put on it, with group members. The elastic band serves as the container in this classroom experiment. Krystal asks her students to stand in a large circle. Once they are in place, she extracts the stretch band from the bag, lays the band in the middle of the circle in a pile, and asks the students to slowly and cautiously step inside, place the band on their lower back, with their hands on either side of the band, and begin walking backward to stretch the band, step by step. This creates a large circular community that is now connected and leans into one shared supportive elastic moving container. It is important to mention that in such an exploration each person's movement, either gentle or dramatic, immediately causes a wave that moves through the entire group. Krystal asks the students one by one to direct the stretch band in a way that moves it in a variety of ways while the other students mirror the movement. Students lift the band over their heads, bend over forward while holding the band, sway side to side with the band around their waists, shake the band by moving their hips back and forth, play with their weight moving the band back and forth all the way, and sometimes just sit down and wiggle the band on the ground.

After the movement with the stretch band concludes, Krystal asks the students to mindfully step out of the stretch band until everyone has done so and then they return to their seats. Krystal asks the students to take out their journals and begin to write reflectively on what it felt like to be contained in the stretch band, and to be part of a movement that became a group movement almost like a wave. You cannot move in the stretch band exercise without affecting one another. Some of the written responses refer to reconnecting to playfulness, trustworthiness, freedom of movement, and experiencing the reminders of childhood in a well-contained and connected space allowing for exploration through the body that might not have happened otherwise. An important lesson for undergraduate expressive arts therapy students who are exploring how they impact and are impacted by others is exemplified and experienced through playing with this simple expanding and retracting band. Furthermore, the students' experiences are being stretched beyond their imaginations.

Regarding other types of containers, Oliver Sacks (2007), a scientific yet artistically talented writer, in his book *Musicophilia*, wrote:

> Music to me has always been a handsome three-dimensional container, a vessel, as real in its way as a scout hut or a cathedral or a ship, with an inside and an outside and subdivided internal spaces. I'm absolutely certain that this "architecture" had everything to do with why music has always exerted such an emotional hold over me.
>
> (p. 160)

Music as a container has some interesting aspects, one of them being that it is an invisible container because we hear and feel it, but we do not see it. We are impacted deeply when we listen to music and we can feel contained by the rhythm, the beat, the melody, the cacophony, and harmony, through and in our bodies, souls, and minds though there is nothing in this container that we can physically grasp in the space around us. This refers to both listening to music and creating music. Leo Tolstoy (1928–1910) has been attributed to have once said, "Music is the shorthand of emotions." Music allows us to contain feelings and, in some experiences, feel more understood than any of our human counterparts can offer verbally.

In a drum circle, Krystal invites each person to choose a hand drum from the middle of the circle. These drums are from many different cultures and each one is described by Krystal and the culture is discussed before the drums are chosen. The drums are not necessarily used in their traditional ways, in the same way that expressive art therapists do not use art supplies, poetry, dance and movement, altars, objects, and words in their traditional ways; imagination is our spine and we use our artistic license.

In the academic setting, Krystal's undergraduate students choose a drum whose sound, shape, or name they find pleasing. Beginning with the student sitting to the right of Krystal, she asks the student to "play a steady and continuous beat." This first invitation is purposely simple and direct. The student begins playing with their fingers or palms and once they have discovered their beat Krystal tells the next student in the circle to become attuned to the vibration of the person who just began drumming and copy what that person is playing. This copying is to indicate to the first student that they are being seen and heard. Once the second student has resonated and mirrored the first beat, they are invited to riff off that beat and start playing a new beat. This ritual is continued over and over throughout the circle, first resonating then riffing, until everyone is playing together after being heard and copied. The community is a circle that is connected through communal beats that each have their own voice but are drumming in an interconnected and new percussive ensemble. While the drummers are playing, Krystal stands up in the middle of the circle at this point and becomes a conductor. She moves her hands and body to guide the musicians to play quietly, loudly, fast, slow, stop, pause, and begin again in the same way the conductor of a symphony works.

When conductor Krystal has given the cue, the music stops, and the musicians become writers. They put down their drums and pick up their pens. They are asked to reflect and respond in writing to each stage of the drumming and the whole experience in its entirety. Some examples and responses are that they feel more connected to the class, they feel more awake versus when they first come to class, they feel free and contained at the same time, and, in some instances, people feel more exposed, they refer to how they feel contained in a human vessel as resonating with the shape of a drum reminding one of a human shape at times. All of these responses are written about in each student's reflective journal. There is something about drumming in particular that invites the expression of emotion in a very physical and meaningful way, which is why drums have been used by a variety of cultures for thousands of years (Rider, 1997). This is a wonderful example of cultural appreciation in music, as opposed to cultural appropriation. Henry David Thoreau (1910) wrote, "If a man does not keep pace with his companions, perhaps it is because he hears a different drummer. Let him step to the music which he hears, however measured or far away" (p. 430). In the drumming circle, it is literally in each participant's hands to decide how they become part of this human and musical container.

Another way that containment can be used in an academic setting sometimes happens online. Containing and community were the focus of an online, one-time check-in session with first and second-year art therapy graduate students. The class took place just after the October 7, 2023, atrocities and war broke out in the Middle East, in which Tamar focused on containment as the topic. Containment was chosen because there was a collective feeling of abandonment and loss of grounding and safety. The students were asked to have paper and writing materials at hand in the first part of the exercise, and Tamar shared with the students that she would be holding up objects in her hand and they would have three minutes to write about each object associatively without lifting their hands from the paper while writing. The objects Tamar held up included: a large clear sparkly plastic bowl, a small basket with a complete removal cover, a dried-out seed pod with the stem still connected, and an orange plastic Kinder Egg® surprise container with a cover that stays connected even when open.

The written expressions to the objects were shared out loud by different students for

the individual containers. Some examples of what the students wrote surprised Tamar and included a raw beginning of a poem about the Kinder

Egg® container that included family memories of joyous occasions and then became somber. The student cried while reading the last part of their poem, becoming very sad, because in Hebrew these containers are called "surprise eggs." The student then wrote that now the word "surprise" is no longer a happy word after what happened on October 7, 2023. Similar to what Ralph Ellison noted, "The act of writing requires a constant plunging back into the shadow of the past where time" hovers ghostlike.

(Ellison, 1963, p. 127)

A different student related to the sparkly clear plastic bowl remembering family parties, in which people brought food to picnics in those kinds of bowls. The student thought that these occasions might happen in the future, even though at the moment, everything felt helpless, isolated, and dark. During collective traumas, and in situations in which people cannot meet in person, be they natural disasters, war, or COVID-19, when people's lives are upended, online platforms themselves can become a container for group participants.

In another example of containment, done in person, Tamar asked 25 expressive therapies graduate students, from all arts languages, including music therapy, drama therapy, art therapy, dance/movement therapy, and bibliotherapy, to bring in single-sized duvet covers. A duvet is a thin sheet-like cover used to envelop thick blankets. The students were asked to move their chairs and tables to the sides of the classroom to create a safe space and setting in which to play, improvise, and carefully move. They were then asked to take their duvet covers and find a place in that space, climb inside the duvet cover, and stand upright and still while getting used to what it feels like to be inside a protected cocoon-like container. Once they felt acclimated to the feeling of being enclosed in their own space, in a room full of other people in their own spaces, they were asked to very gently and slowly move parts of their bodies against the fabric, exploring the gentle pushing and pulling. Some people grabbed the fabric in their fists and pulled it toward their bodies, and others opened their hands and pushed it out, doing similar movements with their knees or feet. They were then invited to do similar movements in the laying down or sitting down. Tamar reminded them that since there were many people in the room, they might find themselves very close to another cocooned being. In this closeness, they could either explore or move away from these meetings. Sometimes when in a lying down position people begin to naturally go into a fetal position or start rolling slowly around the room.

Tamar, as if witnessing an improvisational dance performance, saw a choreography of what seemed like a large group of chrysalises beginning the stage of using their wings to emerge from the inside to the outside. Tamar then invited the students to slowly find a way to exit the closed-in space, in a way that felt right to the process they had been exploring. Some participants immediately emerged while others took quite a long time. Once outside of the duvet cover, they were invited to sit on the fabric on the floor and write in their journals about what it felt like to be on the inside and on the outside. Some examples of responses were that being inside felt comforting and/or womb-like, cave and hibernation associations arose, as opposed to students who felt too closed in, had difficulties with not seeing what was around them, and were challenged by the fabric restricting their movement.

Playing in the duvet cover is quite a somatic and physical manner in which to explore moving between the inside and the outside. The visceral act of feeling oneself push and pull against and with the fabric while not being able to see is very powerful. In the exploration, the metaphor of birth is often mentioned. In general, the use of boxes, masks, and other containers has brought up in both of our groups the associations of both being birthed and giving birth to oneself. The use of the aforementioned containers invites people to explore the beginning of their lives from the inside out, the outside in, and the seams that connect them.

In a world that can feel overwhelming, unsafe, and full of both physical and emotional challenges, wherever you live, containment, and playing with containment through the language of the arts is a true blessing.

Writing Invitations

1 A Word Container: Inside and Outside Words

Find a container to decorate, ornament, and cover with words. A can, a box, a vase, a bottle, an old shoe or boot, a hat, a basket, one you create, perhaps from clay or paper mâché. It can be see-through or not, it can be any shape. You might want to have a cover, you might want to use it as a place for your writing instruments: pens, pencils, etc. Begin the process of collecting printed words from old magazines, journals, newspapers, abandoned books, and old writing that you have written. The words can be from advertisements, articles, stories, poems, or any written material at all. The searching, finding, and cutting or tearing can take time. Put the words in a safe place, perhaps an envelope, and continue to add to them. I prefer a plastic or glass container so I can look at them as I collect them. If you discover a theme arising as you find words, follow the path of that theme; if you do not find a theme continue as is. Once you feel that you are ready to begin adorning your container with the words, start gluing them on. You might want to create negative space in between them, you might glue layer upon layer. This attaching part of the process can also be done over time. Gluing words on the outside AND inside can be meaningful, perhaps words more private go inside, and more disclosing, on the outside. There is no rush! Play with the words, and allow them to be moved to their new home next to new neighbors. What word community is formed? Once you feel that this process is complete, cover the words with a water-based varnish. Art supply stores have many, even white or clear glue works. Use your container, keep it out, and turn it around to find new inspirations, emotions, and combinations. You might want to create a journal after this, that is covered with words that are connected to words that have to do with writing. Tamar has created an altered book covered in this manner.

2   **Self-Guided Imagery and Writing and Artmaking: Writing as Connecting**
Find a comfortable place to sit down, recline, or lie down. Imagine you are walking through a green meadow on a warm, breezy, sunny spring day with a group of friends or family. The wildflowers are abloom, the bees are buzzing as they visit them, and the scent is a blessing to your nose. You begin to get a bit tired, as you have been walking for quite a while. In the distance, you see a large, ancient tree, which is creating a big circle of inviting shade. You walk to this tree and find comfortable positions to enjoy the shadows of the leafy branches. Some of you fall into light naps, some just look quietly at the surroundings. It is silent, no talking is needed to share this moment. One by one you notice shiny, strange sparkles in the grass and wildflowers. Hands reach out to explore. BEADS! You have each found a bead from a broken necklace of someone else who had enjoyed this tree. You hold them in your palms, you roll them between your fingers, and you take them home. Once the day's share journey is complete, you remove the bead and draw or paint a picture of it. You then take a photo of your painting. You all send these photos to one another. You decide as a group to each create a bracelet or necklace by drawing and sculpting, from all of your beads; a group, communal, connecting piece of beaded jewelry in an art form is created in a plethora of ways. This necklace or bracelet is a container of your shared, imagined experience. Write about this: Are you curious about the original owner of the beads? Do you feel more connected to these imagined friends by this connecting and sharing journey? What else is contained in this exploration? Write about whatever this self-guided imagery evoked. These art pieces are shared next time you all get together. Who knows what the next step of this might be…

3   **Your Mask Assemblage**
You will be creating a mask assemblage out of objects that are in your life. Begin to collect objects within your home, current space, or surroundings that identify with your interests current or previous. Once you have finished collecting the objects to represent your interests, begin to assemble them on a flat surface placed in a manner that suits you and is in the shape or form of any kind of mask you can imagine. The background can also be a meaningful part of this process and can be made of any material you choose: objects floating in the water, objects overlapping, on fabric, on a yoga mat, on a mirror, in the grass, on a pillow, on a bed of nails, or even in the palm of your hand. Once you have completed the mask, go to your journal and draw a quick sketch of the outline shape of the mask, and take a photograph of your results and perhaps each step of the way. Write down the names of all of the objects you

chose in detail; be descriptive: texture, shape, color, history, relationship with the objects, and associations and memories. Give the mask a name, and write the name in your journal. Now write what led you to choose these objects and how the placement in this particular manner resonates with your relationship to the mask. Imagine how you would like to keep this mask in your daily life: hung on the wall, placed on a shelf in your bedroom, or hidden away in a time capsule. Feel free to make a new assemblage of materials for your mask each day, once a month, or even once a year as an exploration of the different masks we have in our lives. Engaging with the mask in this manner is reminiscent of personal altar-making; perhaps, this ever-changing mask assembled from objects will become a sacred space to remind you of sacred things about yourself.

4 **Photographing Boxes and Other Containers: From Mundane to Meaningful**

Take a walk in your home and collect some containers, try to have some textural differences, some that you can see through, some not, pasta strainers and colanders, lace, punctured things, broken containers, anything, and everything. Find boxes of different sizes, shapes, and materials. Your home is full of treasures. Even the mundane containers become meaningful now. Take a flashlight and begin to place the objects near or inside one another, and in the boxes. Turn off the lights, and use the flashlight from different angles to cause shadows and lights from and within your boxes. Take lots of photos, play with a mirror as an additional toy, and use more than one flashlight! Perhaps candlelight. Look at the photos and write about each one. Remember that light and dark need each other to exist... In connection to this, chiaroscuro is an Italian term that literally means "light-dark." In paintings, the description refers to clear tonal contrasts which are often used to suggest the volume and modeling of the subjects depicted. Artists who are famed for the use of chiaroscuro include Leonardo da Vinci (Britannica, 2023).

Resources

Books

Written by the drummer of the Grateful Dead, Micky Hart, and colleagues, *Drumming at the Edge of Magic: A Journey into the Spirit of Percussion* shares a passion for drums and other percussion instruments as a vehicle for transformative creative expression. The book was published in 1990 by Harper San Francisco.

Not a Box, is a 2006 children's book written by Antoinette Portis to remind the youngest readers of all of the creative possibilities of a cardboard box. It is published by Harper Collins.

Videos

This November 2015 TED MD talk, *Art Can Heal PTSD Invisible Wounds*, from Melissa Walker shares describes how mask-making can be used to work with veterans, https://www.ted.com/talks/melissa_walker_art_can_heal_ptsd_s_invisible_wounds?language=en

Article

This May 2, 2022, article by R. Lesso discusses Picasso's interest in African Masks after he discovered them as a young man. "Why did Picasso like African Masks?" is published by
The Collector and can be found at: https://www.thecollector.com/why-did-picasso-like-african-masks/.

Places

Visit the National Museum of Mexican Art in Chicago, USA, and look at the Nicho's, the tiny shadow boxes that feature scenes many of El Dia de Los Muertos. This museum had a Nicho making workshop in 2022. Learn more about it on their website: https://nationalmuseumofmexicanart.org/events/nmma-en-casa-nicho-box
https://nationalmuseumofmexicanart.org/artworks.

References

Betensky, M.G. (1995). *What do you see? Phenomenology of therapeutic art expression.* Jessica Kingsley Publishers.

Britannica, T. Editors of Encyclopedia. (2023, November 27). *Chiaroscuro.* Encyclopedia Britannica. https://www.britannica.com/art/chiaroscuro

Demaine, K. (2024). Encountering the mask with undergraduate expressive therapies students: Engaging ritual, dialogue, and reflection. In S. Ridley (Ed.), *Behind the mask: The expressive use of masks across cultures and healing arts* (pp. 105–112). Routledge Publishers.

Einstein, T. (2024). Building trust through mask making in East and West Jerusalem: Developing and exposing, disguising and divulging clinically and in phototherapy training. In S. Ridley (Ed.), *Behind the mask: The expressive use of masks across cultures and healing arts* (pp. 97–104). Routledge Publishers.

Farrell-Kirk, R. (2001). Secrets, symbols, synthesis, and safety: The role of boxes in art therapy. *Journal of the American Art Therapy Association, 39*(3), 88–92.

McNiff, S. (1992). *Art as medicine: Creating a therapy of the imagination.* Shambhala.

Morrison, T. (1992). *Playing in the dark: Whiteness and the literary imagination.* Vintage Books.

No Sweat Shakespeare (n.d.). 'Wear your heart on your sleeves', meaning and context. https://nosweatshakespeare.com/quotes/famous/wear-heart-on-sleeve/

Paris Review. (1963). Interview with Ralph Ellison. In G. Plimpton (Ed.), *Writers at work: The Paris review interviews* (2nd series, book 8). Penguin Books.

Rider, M. (1997). *The rhythmic language of health and disease.* MMB Music, Inc.

Ridley, S. (Ed.) (2024). *Behind the mask: The expressive use of masks across cultures and healing arts.* Routledge.

Sacks, O. (2007). *Musicophilia: Tales of music and the brain.* Knopf.

Smith, Z. (2003). *White teeth,* Knopf Doubleday Publishing Group.

Thoreau, H. D. (1910). *Walden.* Thomas Y. Crowell and Co.

Zechner, S. (2016, July 19). 10 Fascinating cultural masks from around the world. *Western Union.* https://www.westernunion.com/blog/en/cultural-masks-of-the-world/

Chapter 9

Letters, Notes, and Handwriting

Krystal Leah Demaine and Tamar Reva Einstein

Welcome Mat: This chapter will call upon the lost art of letter writing. The sentiment and value of handwriting will be addressed. This will include lamenting the past kinds of writings while comparing them to the present technology-based forms of written communication. Nostalgic stories and writing rituals are shared. Goldberg (1986) wrote, "Handwriting is more connected to the movement of the heart." The concept of writing as heart-based, done by hand, is a connecting of two parts of our bodies and feelings woven together (p. 8).

The Lost Art of Letter Writing

In this age of ever-changing, fast-paced technological development, receiving handwritten notes and letters has become rare. Emails, direct messaging, texting, and so forth have become the norm. It seems that we less and less even scribble handwritten "to do" notes to ourselves, let alone write to others. Due to the nostalgic love of handwriting, museums have even had exhibitions addressing the longing for this human handmade mark-making. The Morgan Library & Museum in Manhattan, New York City, USA, featured 140 rare notes, manuscripts, sketches, signatures, and letters; it was just a taste of the extensive 100,000 document collection belonging to Brazilian historian and author Pedro Corrêa do Lago (2018). Some of the treasures were penned by Albert Einstein, Leon Trotsky, and Rene Magritte. The exhibition included Michelangelo's schematic design for a marble order for one of his works; a letter from Trotsky to Kahlo during the unraveling of their love affair; and a letter from Oscar Wilde requesting a seat reservation from Brahm Stoker at the theater (Ferro, 2018). Writer, Emily Dickinson (1986) sensed letters as enduring, stating that, "A letter always seemed to me like immortality because it is the mind alone without corporeal friend" (p. 752).

The Fountain House Gallery in Hell's Kitchen, New York, showed an exhibition titled "The Strangers Project," which featured 800 handwritten stories each written on a single piece of paper hung on twine with a single clothespin; suggesting that handwriting is not dead (Lockwood, 2019). The project curator

DOI: 10.4324/9781003391876-10

Brandon Doman started collecting letters from strangers in 2009 by asking them what it is like to be you. Doman believes that everyone has a story to tell and he wants people to be able to share their stories by writing them down in their handwriting. Now he posts where he is going to be on Instagram and he collects handwritten letters in person. Much to his surprise, Doman now has 85,000, and growing, stories collected so far ("The Strangers Project," n.d.).

For over 20 years, Tamar has been giving her students handwritten feedback on their papers in rubber-stamped envelopes. After completing her doctoral degree, she began teaching graduate students; the first time she received 75 papers she needed to respond to, she felt an innate need to respond by writing a brief handwritten letter for each one. Once she read the papers and wrote the letters on small pieces of lined paper, she found envelopes in the art supply store that were the same miniature size as her letters. She excitedly placed each small letter in an individual envelope, sealed it, handwrote the name of the student on the front of the envelope, and left it on the table in the classroom. The next morning, when she saw the pile of envelopes with their names on them, she went to her rubber stamp collection and chose a lizard stamp; lizards being the animal she looks up to because of their ability to transform. She then turned the envelopes over and hand-stamped each envelope, both on the front and back with lizards climbing all over the envelopes. The lizard stamping has now become a tradition. Luckily for Tamar, her colleagues allow her this unique way of responding to her students versus the traditional way of writing on the margins of students' typed and double-spaced formal papers.

The interest in the lost art of handwriting in general, which is connected to letter writing, refers to the end of the era in which each person's unique mark, penmanship, and writing style, have slowly become extinct. We, and many of our colleagues and friends, grieve this intimate personal and one-of-a-kind written artifact. Handwriting has become an artifact. We treasure old handwritten letters, historical family documents, birth announcements, handwritten eulogies, and notes to self, sometimes written on napkins, inside matchbooks, on the back of photographs, and sometimes in leatherbound travel logs. Letters were written by hand to lovers, family members, friends, or professional colleagues. Authors sent their handwritten book manuscripts in large manila hand-addressed envelopes to their editors; with many stamps affixed to the exterior. Before electronic copy machines were invented, authors placed a piece of carbon paper between two pieces of paper as they wrote their manuscript; this produced two copies of their handwritten book. The author kept the carbon copy while the original was sent to the publisher. We are part of the tribe of people who greatly lament "the handwritten." We still handwrite and appreciate receiving handwritten letters and notes.

Handwriting and Handwritten Letters

Before the sudden death of Krystal's father in 2018, he handed her a copy of her original birth certificate folded in half in a brown manila envelope, with her name handwritten in her father's handwriting on the outside. Krystal could not have known how sacred this seemingly mundane moment was at the time. It is a strange dichotomy that his last written object to Krystal before he died was one pronouncing her very birth. Krystal always had a deep curiosity and love of her parents' handwriting and saved many handwritten notes and letters, but this one has a special place in her heart. Krystal connects the handwriting to the visceral memory of her father touching the pen with which her name was written and the envelope where the birth certificate was kept. The circle of life connection is very powerful in this story. Krystal will never forget her father's handwriting.

From an intergenerational perspective on Krystal's father's side of the family, there is another important letter-connected story. Krystal's paternal grandparents left behind a treasure trove of love letters that Krystal has documented. These were written while they were courting each other. Her grandfather's letters are poetic in their language and spare no metaphoric gems. Her grandfather, Robert, compared receiving letters from Esther, her grandmother, to "Any better tonic for the system" and as, "mean as a humble bee that's away from his honey. Now I'm a changed person who sees a new light breaking forth" (R. Bloom, personal communication, August 30, 1938).

Concerning how long people had to wait to receive mail in the 1930s, compared to how quickly we receive email nowadays, Robert writes: "As hungry as I was when I got home today, I just had to read your letter before preparing myself to replenish my stomach" (R. Bloom, personal communication, August 16, 1938). It seems like waiting so long for a letter made them more sacred, and meaningful, and provided us with much-needed soul food.

At the age of 12, when Tamar and her family moved from Manhattan to Jerusalem, letter writing was the only mode of communication to connect with family and friends in the 1970s. Tamar's family did not have a telephone in their apartment for the first four years of living there. There was, however, a public phone in the common area of their apartment building. Yet, making phone calls was virtually impossible as phone use time was pre-scheduled. All those who lived in the same apartment building had a specific time block for their phone time. Letter writing, therefore, became the dominant form of communication for Tamar and her family to contact the life they had left behind. No pun intended, but it is important to note here, that before the invention of telephones, computers, text messages, airplanes, trains, cars, and the internet, and now drones; letter writing was always the only form of communication between people. Furthermore, those letters were delivered by horse, camel, donkey, and sometimes pigeons or other animals indigenous to where the writer lived. Mail delivery carriers literally delivered no matter what! As the US Postal Service motto proclaimed, "Neither rain, nor snow, nor sleet, nor hail shall keep the postmen from their appointed rounds" (Varano, 2015).

The most popular form of written international communication came in the form of lightweight airmail letters known as aerograms. Aerograms were made of a piece of long, rectangular, pale blue colored paper, with pre-glued tabs on the sides, and vaguely seen lines in certain places that served as directions to show you where to fold, glue, and mail. Aerograms were like magical pieces of origami where the letter, when folded, became its own envelope that must be folded in one certain way for it to work; and once you received the letter, there was a specific way you had to open it so that you would not accidentally split the letter in half. The aerogram was pre-stamped and purchased only at the post office, with the correct postage according to the country of destination. Tamar waited with bated breath for her aerograms to arrive and could immediately recognize from the exterior handwriting who it was from, before even looking at the return address. Tamar was motivated to immediately answer the letters like an ongoing conversation.

As a budding teenager, Tamar wrote many aerograms to her friends and loved ones in the States. It might be important to mention that such air mail did not move as quickly in the 1970s as it does today and it took quite a while, at least several weeks to mail and receive these letters; hence the reason we refer to this as snail mail. In case of emergencies, telegrams were sent. Tamar has kept two type-written telegrams that were sent to her in Israel from her US family to celebrate her Bat Mitzvah. Nowadays, while Tamar communicates regularly with many of the same people through free international texting, email, and online video plat-forms, she misses handwriting and the memories attached to each person's unique, though sometimes illegible writing. Tamar does appreciate how one can connect over thousands of miles immediately via the technology of the current era.

Did you know that noted painter, Vincent Van Gogh, according to the Van Gogh Museum (n.d.), was also a voracious letter writer, composing more than 2,000 letters? Among these letters, mostly written to his brother who kept a vast amount, some were written to his sister and others as well. Within the letters, he often included rough renderings of his painting ideas. Further, he only signed the letters with his first name, just as he did his paintings which started because living in France, the local people could not pronounce his last name properly. One can visit the Van Gogh Museum in Amsterdam to read and gaze upon the riveting collection of letters to and mostly from the artist himself.

The slow fade out and diminishing of writing and receiving handwritten letters has created for both authors an enormous appreciation of saved handwritten notes, documents, and letters from family and friends. This personal connection through the flowing ink of bygone fountain pens is reminiscent of the intergener-ational blood that flows through our family's veins. It carries our DNA, cultures, told and untold stories, and most importantly allows us to share this with the next generation. As Japanese Writer, Haruki Murakami (2000) so eloquently stated

How wonderful it is to be able to write someone a letter! To feel like convey-ing your thoughts to a person, to sit at your desk and pick up a pen, to put your thoughts into words like this is truly marvelous.

(p. 86)

One might add to Murakami's statement, how wonderful it is to also receive such a letter.

Signatures and Autographs

Signatures and autographs, like handwritten letters, at one time, carried important information including proof of identity and legitimized contractual agreements like marriage licenses, divorces, loans, house deeds, and other binding contracts. These days signatures are often done digitally. In certain cultures and religions, the signing of documents in the presence of witnesses was enough to ensure that that document was binding. Now, we are left wondering what will happen to the importance of any signature used for legal, moral, cultural, and financial paperwork in the age of technology that now includes artificial intelligence. In the same way that we once looked at photographs for evidence and proof in news articles, for example, photos and signatures can be easily manipulated by and with the use of artificial intelligence by humans. Perhaps the signature is the last symbol of handwritten legitimacy that is disappearing and becoming questionable because of how easy it is to tamper with.

Another aspect of signatures is the emotional meaning that they carry. Some people keep photographs in their wallets, that are hand-signed and dated on the back, or with messages written. Historical ancestral documents, as mentioned before, are sometimes treasured because of the signatures. There are even people who have family or beloved's names, and sometimes signatures in their original handwriting tattooed on their bodies as a process known as memorial tattoos, especially after someone passes away (Steadman et al., 2023).

Some people collect signed and autographed objects. For example, first edition books signed by authors, sports or music memorabilia, and let us not forget about signed artwork at auctions, which has become an astronomically lucrative financial market that ironically often is of paintings created by people who died alone, sick, or starving. For example, Vincent Van Gogh's paintings sold for millions of dollars after he died in 1890 while he was poor and suffering from multi-layered mental and physical illnesses (Arnold, 2004). Van Gogh's *Orchard with Cypress* painting sold in 2022 at Christie's Auction in New York for 117.2 million dollars (Burgess, 2023). It is the artist's signature that may give the work unparalleled monetary value.

Adults and children alike can become obsessed with collecting autographs. Some notable people, movie stars, politicians, famous writers, musicians, and famous chefs, are followed around and asked for their autographs. But, once again, because of technology, now those famous people are asked to take a selfie with the fan. This generation does not even know how to sign on the dotted line (LoRusso, 2020).

If we were going to enter a time machine and go back centuries to when etiquette was highly proclaimed, we would see that signatures were very important in reserving an opportunity to have a meeting for what we now call a date. These dates often happened at social dances. If you are coming with us in the time machine, please don't forget your dance card!

Social dances in the 18th to 20th centuries required that women be invited to the ball beforehand and receive a dance card as part of their invitation. This card had the names of the dances, a polka, a waltz, a galop, a mazurka, and a quadrille in order on the program. There was an empty line next to the name of each dance to leave room for a man to write his name in pencil to save that specific dance for that particular woman. For example, Lord Stripey Pants III could reserve his polka dance with Lady Crinoline II.

Sometimes the woman attached the card to her wrist or turned the card into a fan so she could see the names of the men more easily, or potentially fan themselves when they got hot. We must not forget the ritual when encountering the woman, the man had to step a few feet away from the woman, bow, and then the woman had to bow reciprocally and then the dance could begin. Women were completely forbidden from choosing male dance partners. The dance card, even though written in pencil, served as a signed contract. It was the man's autograph and signature that made the dance card real and that real signature could not be broken. Sometimes the men were naughty and chose to dance the polka with women whom they had just danced the quadrille leaving the man whose name was written on the card angered. Because it was considered improper to dance with someone not written on your card, the abandoned woman would have to sit it out on her own (American Antiquarian Society, 2007). You might have heard someone saying the adage: "[So and so]'s dance card is full." This adage is directly connected to Victorian dance cards and meant that a woman's dance card was full of names and had no room for new suitors. Or as we might say now, sorry, I'm already taken!

Another form of signing objects is the love token. According to the Love Token Society (2012), a love token is a coin, usually a dime, that has been smoothed flat on one side and then hand-engraved. The smoothed side of the coin is then hand-monogrammed elaborately and engraved by a male suitor with his initials and given to his darling to court her. The young woman remembered the suitor when she looked at the love token. There is a specific set of guidelines for the creation of these love coins; the coin must be a dime and current of the time, and the initials hand etched.

Penmanship

When we were in grade school in the 1960s and 1980s respectively, we were required to take a class called penmanship. There were special notebooks for these classes that were designed exclusively to help us learn how to write upper-case and lower-case letters. Once we learned how to print and write our letters, everyone learned how to write in script also known as cursive handwriting. This flowing way of writing, in which the letters are connected, is no longer taught in the school system, as far as we know.

An *NPR* news report (Martin & Kaur, 2022) cited that cursive writing and reading requirements were cut from the Common Core curriculum in the United States in 2010, making it a non-required standard for academic learning. The report noted that America's founding documents are written in cursive limiting its future readers. Perhaps in the future, there will be graduate studies in cursive writing and reading, as it dwindles as a long-lost practice; in the same way that languages that are becoming extinct are now offered for study in the United States.

We both find beauty and artistry in cursive handwriting. Tamar has kept a copy of her grandmother's travel journal from what was her first trip to the Middle East in the late 1940s. The journal was written in cursive English which was not her mother tongue, it was Polish. When she moved to America as a young woman from Poland and was learning English, she was taught to write in cursive and printed English. The script from the travel journal was like a beautiful artwork; it is breathtaking. This beauty of handwriting is not taught, or practiced as much as it once was, and its essence is at risk of becoming obsolete. We wonder at what age people need to learn how to write their signatures, and if learning how to sign something is relevant anymore. Sometimes people don't even need to sign when they use their credit cards in the grocery store, or other places because there are machines that accept your cell phone app, your fingerprint, or face recognition as a form of payment linked to your account, as technology moves forward.

Envelopes, Stationary, and Stamps

Selecting envelopes and paper or stationery that we write on was once a common practice among letter writers. There are still paper stores where shelves of extremely beautiful paper and envelopes that you can select as well as matching sets of notecards with envelopes and sometimes a matching pen are found. Stationary envelopes and paper come in different thicknesses, colors, materials, finishes, and even scents. We have noticed as of late that there seems to be a resurgence of shops that specialize in paper, writing implements, and all things connected to the lost art of letter writing. Nowadays, on special occasions, rites of passage, perhaps weddings or other significant celebrations, some people still choose special paper; sometimes they will handwrite the envelopes in calligraphy or embossed with metallic stamps. However, many people are instead choosing digital invitations and announcements for both technological and environmental reasons. For example, some people might print invitations on seed-embedded recycled paper, not only protecting trees but also planting new seedlings.

Oftentimes stationery and envelopes accompanied one another along with essential and oftentimes special postage stamps. Krystal still purchases all of her stamps at her local post office and in doing so, asks the teller behind the counter if they have any "unique or cool" stamps in stock. Stamps often commemorate special historical moments, artists, writers, heroes and heroines, seasons, animals, social and political movements, and holidays. *Philately* refers to the study of stamps and one who collects stamps may refer to themselves as a *philatelist* or more simply put, a stamp collector. According to the Stanley Gibbons website (n.d.), stamp collecting is one of the most popular hobbies worldwide and has been since stamps were introduced in 1840. Collectors save stamps that are used, unused, postmarked, and designed with both common and fine art themes from across the world. Krystal's mother used the age-old technique of steaming the stamps off the envelopes, over a bowl of boiling water, creating a collage of vintage stamps from the correspondence between her paternal grandparents.

Along with paper and pens, there were and still are other writing paraphernalia that writers use and love, and some even collect. For example, manual pencil sharpeners sometimes attached to a table or a wall, ink wells and fountain pens, envelopes, postage stamp sponges, postage stamp dispensers, wax envelope seals, embossers, rubber stamps, stickers including personalized address stickers, bookmarks, ex-libris, carbon paper, and letter openers. When Tamar was a very young child, her grandfather used to let her open his mail with his red plastic Fuller Brush® (n.d.) man letter opener. Tamar recalls it to be so exciting to open these letters so carefully and precisely. As an adult, Tamar found a similar relic at a vintage shop, though not the same red color, but just as special. Tamar keeps her Fuller Brush® letter opener on her desk where she can keep it at all times.

Passing Notes

Krystal has kept all of the handwritten notes she and her best friend passed to each other in middle school in the late 1980s. These notes were written on pieces of lined paper torn from their notebooks and sometimes included drawings and plans to meet up after school or to go to the movies on the weekend, secret ramblings of feeling bored in gym class and knowing that her friend could relate. Occasionally, the notes were folded in a triangular shape, that could fit in the palm of one's hand, the folding technique was called a football. Some students in school would flick their paper footballs across the classroom for their friends to catch, but Krystal and her friend passed each other the notes in the hallway to not get caught participating in the taboo note-passing act. This note-passing method is unfamiliar to Tamar who in her class used to roll up notes lengthwise, slide them inside an inkless pen, and blow into the pen tube to shoot the note across the room like a spitball.

For some students note passing is a form of rebellion, and in the classroom when you are always the passer and not the recipient of the note, it can feel isolating. In Krystal's undergraduate courses, she encourages note and letter passing as a form of communication and response to in-class activities, as previously discussed in the letter writing section, including the mask discussed in Chapter 8 and musical life reviews covered in Chapter 1. Krystal believes from her own childhood experience that passing notes encourages communication, expressing oneself through writing, and playful creative connection which is a goal she encourages in all of her undergraduate expressive arts therapy students.

An article in the *Higher Education Times* (Kinsella & Kaye, 2021) also supports and even encourages note passing in the higher education classroom, suggesting that the act helps support communication and feeling connected to peers. Especially in online classes, where students can pass private digital messages, reactions in the form of emojis, and reflections that might help students better understand the subject matter.

While there is a time when note passing may be appropriate, such as in reflection of a student presentation where all students are passing a note to that one presenter, it can otherwise be a distraction. As educators of the future therapists of the world, we need to cultivate a sense of belonging, inclusion, and presence in our classrooms. When students become distracted, isolated, or perhaps non-participatory for other reasons it can disrupt the flow of the classroom process and the clinical skills that the students must cultivate.

There is a difference between intentionally planned activities such as focused note passing in response to specific activities and being distracted. In years past, one might doodle or work on other assignments rather than paying attention to what was happening in class. Today, however, there is an ever more present and all too easy distraction in the form of cell phones, tablets, and laptops. Yet one cannot be a therapist with a phone in hand. For this reason, we both require students' cell phones and laptops to be put away during class time. As therapists, we have the enormous responsibility of practicing presence with our clients, active witnessing, and facilitation, and we must be present. Starting with our behavior in the class classroom is how we demonstrate this essential clinical skill of presence with clients. When people have laptops open, perhaps paying bills and doing other work, they are not present in class. Can you imagine being in therapy and your therapist is multi-tasking looking at their cell phone the whole time? In our practice, it is important to be completely present with the senses, perhaps senses that we were not aware we needed; such as looking at body language, listening to the spaces between words, paying attention to people's eye moments, and eye gaze, and in expressive arts therapy being highly aware of how the arts are being utilized. The passing notes of the olden days are very different than what happens today in graduate or undergraduate school.

We have observed that staying connected deeply to one thing can be challenging for people; though it is expected of us from society. As academics and mothers, we have been taught that multi-tasking in this day and age is often considered a highly revered talent. However, our lives become scattered when we are overly multi-tasking, being mindful is indigenous to being a therapist.

Note-writing and texting can be tempting and addictive, and we do get a dopamine boost with the social reward of sending and receiving (Haynes, 2018). Because we are teaching expressive arts therapy, we need to model behavior; our methods of teaching require group participation and all of the senses to be awake, aware, connected, and cross-connected weaving a spider web across and through the circle, as we teach with students sitting in a circle. We understand that our students are so used to using their phones and relying on them, for a variety of different reasons, but we need them to be present.

In group therapy, we have asked our clients to put cell phones in a basket at the beginning of the session to keep them focused. There are enormous benefits to this technology of being able to connect with people when we need them, however, there are also downfalls. Like everything in life, we need to find a healthy balance when using any kind of communication be they handwritten notes, cell phones, tablets, or laptops.

Emergency Situations, Texting, and Connecting

Some situations are unique and carry a very heavy need for connection, sharing, venting, and hearing a loved one's voice. Sometimes we need our phones and immediate ways to contact people when they can be life-saving or help avoid life-threatening situations, and other times those modes of communication are not allowed or available. There are also places where it is considered inconsiderate and perhaps unsafe for use; such as, in waiting rooms in hospitals and clinics, places of worship, or on airplanes.

In a casual conversation in December 2023, between Tamar and other expressive therapists, a discussion arose about how soldiers communicate with their loved ones during a war. While soldiers may be allowed to bring their cell phones into the war zone, there are dangers inherent in their usage. As we all know, cell phones track information such as one's location. Thus, to allow soldiers to communicate with their families, some new, yet old-fashioned, creative solutions have been invented. The first creative solution involves paper and envelopes, which are handed out to soldiers to write letters during their very short breaks. The letters are collected by a soldier who takes the letters beyond the border to be distributed to the addressees by a mail carrier or by hand. These are handwritten letters with hand-addressed envelopes. The second creative solution is that after the soldier hand writes the letters on the paper, their superior photographs the handwritten letters, crosses the border, and then digitally sends photos of the handwritten letters to the recipients. This harkens back to the days of WWI and WWII when carrier pigeons were used to transport behind the lines. This has made the authors wonder if we will see a resurgence of handwritten letter writing, note writing, and note passing in people's personal written script in the future. Ironically, this mailing of letters in this old-fashioned way now must be done because of security reasons. It is important to mention that sometimes the use of a cell phone for tracking is extremely helpful and useful; for example, people with dementia, children who may be in danger, parents who want to track their teenager, and those who might be frail or need help. Communication has changed over centuries, but our main interest is that no matter what kind of writing one is doing to communicate, writing is important and meaningful in many different situations. We believe that communication through writing continues to be a basic human need.

Chain Letters and Pen Pals

Did you know that June 1 is National Pen Pal Day in the United States (National Day Calendar, n.d.)? According to the Pen Pal Community Blog (Maud, 2022), the friendly handwritten letter exchanges termed pen pal writing came into play in 1936 when a student letter exchange organization gave it the name. The original term was *pen-friend*, which first appeared in 1919 with the same connotation. Historically, pen pals were designed for relationships that were purely written exchanges wherein the letter writers might never actually meet, and oftentimes lived thousands of miles apart.

There is also a practice of having pen pals with people who have been incarcerated. There are a variety of different organizations that can assign an incarcerated person a pen pal from a non-prison setting. According to Wire of Hope's Prison Pen Pal Program (n.d.), incarcerated individuals who have a pen pal are 60% less likely to have recurring offenses once released from prison. According to the Prison Letters Project (Bazelon & Lennon, 2022), these types of correspondences with incarcerated individuals have helped exonerate the wrongly accused and supported the resolution of issues with the criminal justice system. Receiving letters in prison can help isolated and incriminated people feel connected, cared for, and heard, which is very important for a person's mental health.

When Krystal was in high school English class, she distinctly remembers the pen pal assignment being introduced as a method of practicing formal letter writing and building exchanges with peers of her age from other school districts. Her class was asked to identify three other high schools anywhere in the country and send a letter directed to: "Any student in the high school English class." Being the 1990s, and a huge Grunge Alternative Rock fan, Krystal chose schools on the West coast of the United States where her favorite bands Nirvana, Weezer, and Alice in Chains hailed from, and therefore sent a letter to a high school in Washington, one in California, another in Arizona. Since her search predated the advent of the internet and Google Maps, she used the school library's atlas to find some unique-sounding town names to send her letters to. Of the three schools she contacted, one boy at a high school in Costa Mesa, California, replied to her. Krystal and the boy maintained the writing practice three times each until it fizzled out.

As a young girl, while Tamar was in Hebrew school in Manhattan, she was assigned a pen pal who lived in Israel and was also an English speaker. They began writing to each other regularly for over a few years. When Tamar moved to Israel, their mothers decided they should meet each other in person, which they did. When they met in person, the connection they developed as pen pals dissipated between them, however, their mothers became extremely close friends. In this case, the pen pal relationship moved up a generation and stayed strong and steady for over 40 years.

We would like to take this moment to reflect on a short cautionary tale about writing to people in other countries, where English is not their mother tongue, and one might find oneself in the word quicksand of Google Translate or autocorrect. In this real-life example, Tamar's son and his classmates, in the early 2000s, were invited to a peace celebration in Germany and to stay with a German family in the village. All of the parents were asked to communicate with each other by email before the trip occurred. It was suggested that English should be used as the common language; however, English was not the mother tongue of almost 90% of this group of people who mostly spoke Hebrew, Arabic, or German. Because Tamar's mother tongue was English, she was sent emails from some of the other parents who could not understand the English in these emails because the families were using the Google translate app where many hilarious mistakes were made. In one of the emails to "Dear Johnny," Google Translate replaced the word "Dear" with "Expensive," which still today makes Tamar and her son laugh almost uncontrollably. Henceforth they continue to call Johnny, "Expensive Johnny." The moral of the story is, please, we caution you, be very careful when translating your typed letters into other languages, and run them by people who speak the native tongue before pressing the send button.

One area of writing that both of us, as authors, readers, and writers, have found to be slightly disconcerting is chain letters. We have found that being pressured to forward a letter is tormenting. One is not really given a choice whether or not to forward the letter. One is in turn handed a request to send along the same letter to many other people, or else… We would like to be asked ahead of time to be a part of the chain, not forced into it. But seriously, there is a unique dichotomy to chain letters; for some, chain letters may like being involved in a wonderful growing community; and for others, it feels like being forced into a community that may not be of interest to that person. Chain letters continue to persist and for the most part have gone into the digital realm, via email, making it very easy to forward your letter with just a click of a button if you choose.

Letting Go: Letters as Releasing Rituals

Letter writing is also used to express and release feelings, thoughts, and emotions. There are rituals that people have adopted, invented, continued, and practiced that are referred to as releasing rituals. We practice these releasing rituals through writing in groups, in academia, and personally. These rituals are connected to the four elements in that when releasing things written on paper, one may let go of them by or through water, fire, earth, and air. These rituals may include burning them by fire, immersing them in water, burying them in the ground, and allowing the papers to be taken by the wind.

Within an expressive arts therapy group of adult victims of terror attacks, Tamar developed an arts-based exercise in which both writing and expressing anger were connected. These creations came about after many victims wished to physically express their frustration and anger. The participants were invited to write feelings that were hard to say aloud on small slips of paper. Then they were given clay and Tamar showed them how to make balls from the clay from two halves, before the halves were connected, the notes were put inside. The balls were smoothed into small round clay spheres and left to dry until the next session. Next time, Tamar and the clients all walked downstairs and outside, facing a wall of the building. They were invited to feel the clay ball, now hardened, between their hands, and when ready to throw it with all their might against the wall. One by one, in turns that were not pre-planned, the balls were hurled, smashed, and the written notes strewn about. Some participants made sounds, yelled, cursed, or threw silently. All of the participants reported that they were sated by the act. Then, the notes were randomly collected, as were some pieces of the shards of broken clay. The words were read aloud, not necessarily the ones the participant wrote, but the ones they collected, and a group poem was written from these words. The shards were used in future artworks. In the closing discussion that day the participants expressed feeling many diverse emotions from exhaustion to relief. The word "freeing" came up, and many spoke about how hard it is to really, somatically release anger. This was done with other groups afterward and always had similar results, of a feeling of freedom. Once, Tamar added a pinata, creating then breaking it as a group and collecting the words that had been inside. Then writing was done.

Another place where we use writing for letting go is in hospice work, in which Tamar was immersed for 27 years. Hospice is a rich and complex world of celebrating the end of life, being witness to suffering, and walking the last path with people. One of these people, a woman who had bravely decided not to receive more treatment after years of ups and downs with cancer, worked through many creative forms of expressive arts therapies with Tamar for more than a year. The culmination of this process, when she began to feel death approaching faster, was letter writing to all of her siblings who lived abroad. Tamar offered writing paper, pens, company, chewing gum to help her swallow, and silent witnessing as she wrote.

The client requested to make a short video that would accompany the letters in which she said goodbye to her family in Mexico, while she was dying. The client and the hospital both provided informed consent. Once all the farewell letters were written, put in hand-addressed envelopes, and sealed, Tamar placed them in a large white envelope with the video. Tamar was given a detailed written explanation of how and when to mail these: after the patient died, by airmail, and from the post office nearby. This was all done at the right time, as she quickly deteriorated; Tamar and the staff took turns holding her hand, with prayers playing from a CD player, as we knew she wanted, as she passed. The envelope was mailed as requested. It felt strange, after so many intimate months together, to send off these sacred letters not knowing much about who, when, and how they would be received.

In arts and verbal grief support groups Krystal co-led with a grief counselor for adults and through a hospice organization, there was a process in the last 30 minutes of the 2-hour-long group that started with each person handwriting a letter on a piece of paper to the person they knew who had died. The adults participated in this group to explore and process the loss of a dear one. Once each person finished writing the letter, they all went outside to the back of the building where a hand-made metal bowl, made by the counselor, meant for burning things rested on the ground. In a ritual created by Krystal and her co-counselor to use fire to let go of things, one by one, the participants walked over to the large copper bowl where they were invited to briefly say something silently or audibly before the facilitators struck the match and touched the letter with the flame. Then, the participant placed the letter that was aflame into the bowl and watched it turn from paper to ashes; ashes to ashes. The letter-burning ritual is a reminder of the unsaid words, the things that are let go, and the wish to send a note back into the energy of the universe. Universally in rituals of rites of passage that include fire, the keeper of the ritual, the fire keeper, be they a facilitator, shaman, priest, or rabbi is often the one who begins the fire and contains it.

After finding the burning bowl ritual experience meaningful, Krystal decided to include it as part of her undergraduate therapeutic writing course. The ritual with the students was done at the end of the 15-week semester, with the same idea of a rite of passage that symbolized the end of something important, but not necessarily grief. Krystal asks her students to compose two handwritten letters in the classroom. She begins by handing out a single piece of paper and an envelope to each student. She then asks the students to write their permanent mailing address on the front of the envelope and on the piece of paper to write a letter to their "future self" telling them something valuable, important, or meaningful that they want to take with them as the course ends. When the students finish writing their letters to themselves, they are asked to fold the letter, place it in the envelope, seal it up, and hand it to Krystal who keeps it in her office for a full year until she mails them.

As a next step, Krystal hands out a faintly photocopied piece of paper of natural plants from the college campus, including leaves, berries, and twigs arranged in different ways. The pictures of the plants on the paper symbolize memories of the college campus which is in nature. Krystal could have chosen to use an online image, but the importance of this ritual propelled her to invent a creative process in which she collects nature objects from around the campus and places them on the Xerox machine in different patterns and positions, she prints out a few of the assemblages and allows students to choose them. Imagine a glass Xerox plate being covered with seeds and leaves, almost becoming its own nature altar. Once the students have chosen a piece of paper, they are invited to write a letter to another person. This can be an imaginary or real, living or dead person to whom they have something important to say. It is very important to note that Krystal explains to her students that this letter, message, or note will never reach this person in real life. Once students finish writing this second letter to "the other," Krystal asks them to fold the letter and follow her outside, to the beach across the street. Krystal carries her small two-foot-tall chiminea, which is a portable outdoor fireplace made of terracotta clay, and she places it in the sand on the beach. Similar to her grief support group, Krystal asks the students to come to the chiminea one by one and invites her students to either audibly or silently say, "I release this and let it go." She then strikes her match, lights the letter, and asks the student to place it in the chiminea. During this process there is a silent camaraderie among the students, as they witness one another and seem mesmerized by the flame, the smoke, and the words spoken by their peers. Once all of the letters have been burned, some tears shed, and a few hugs exchanged, the group releases the ashes from the chiminea which are carried away into the wind. All of the emotions, tears, and hugs are also carried away in the wind. This is an example of how what we learn in our clinical groups gets translated and passed forward to our students in our classes, sometimes years later. This chiminea carries and holds hundreds of written stories and secrets like all ritual objects.

Other rituals of letting go are prevalent in many parts of the world as traditions and rituals be they religious, spiritual, artistic, or personal. For example, in Judaism, on the second day of Rosh Hashanah, the Jewish New Year, there is a letting go ritual called Tashlich, where people say a special prayer as they let go of the crumbs in their pocket, to symbolize letting go of the year and welcoming the new year. According to tradition, this release of crumbs must be done only in running water. Tamar has personally reinvented this ritual for herself in different ways, over the years, both alone and with friends, sometimes writing notes of things they would like to change for the new year and burying those notes in potted plants in the garden. Sometimes floating the notes in bowls of water with flower petals watching the paper slowly disintegrate over the holiday, and then using the water to water the plants in her garden. Sometimes writing the notes on very thin paper, illustrating them with images, leaving them in the backyard under the fig tree, and letting them be taken away by the wind. Tamar has never done a fire ritual for Rosh Hashanah but was invited to a winter solstice celebration years ago in which the host had a large ceramic bowl on their patio. The guests were asked to write small notes of things they would like to leave behind from the year. And as the party progressed people slowly and casually wrote and burned their letters in the ceramic bowl at their own pace; quietly and not as a group, but being witnessed and held by the group. For Tamar, the process affirmed and was reminiscent of ancient rituals of rites of passage, which often include letting go of the past to move forward. The four elements; earth, wind, water, and fire, can all be connected to writing notes and letters in rituals, rites of passage, transformation, and letting go.

Writing Invitations

1 **Writing about Things You Accidentally Encounter: Making Magic from a Mess**
   While wandering, meandering, walking, visiting places, look down, look up, look sideways for a moment, and see if you might have stumbled upon a magical mess that you can write about.
   For example:

- A lost doll, shoe, or scarf in the street.
- A pile of wet old photos near the garbage in the rain.
- A broken chair, planter, old building materials, or a torn flag, precariously placed on an upstairs patio or roof.
- A note on a wall that a watch, piece of jewelry, and wallet has been found with a phone number to retrieve the item.
- An abandoned, book, notebook, magazine, or newspaper on a bench left open at a page, or turned and crumpled.
- A balloon, plastic bag, shiny streamer, soccer ball, or strings caught randomly in tree branches.
- Broken computers, vacuum cleaners, and furniture left on sidewalks in pieces.
- A pile of old clothes placed on a wall or fence in an unruly and unkempt manner.
- Personal documents overflowing in cardboard boxes left near a recycling bin and strewn on the ground.
- Boxes of empty broken and whole glass wine and beer bottles left in an empty lot of wildflowers.
- An abandoned building destroyed and lying in pieces.

Write about what these objects conjure for you, what are these grouped or individual messes? To whom might they have belonged? What might you turn them into as you write about them; what magical stories can they become? Maybe take a photo to view at home so that you can look at it while you write. What spoke to you as you discovered the image; is it a metaphor for you? What emerges as you write? Perhaps make a collage or any other piece of art from the emotions and images that arise with your writing. How can you create magic from a mess?

2 Writing Notes that You Never Dared to Write in School

Imagine yourself now in your middle school or high school classroom. Close your eyes and remember all of the people sitting there and think of all of the moments when you didn't dare pass a note but wanted to. What would you have written in that note? Who would you give that note to? You are even allowed to write that note to teachers. Now, write that note, be as specific as possible, trying to remember the person's name, where they sat, and what you always wanted to express but couldn't then; now is your chance! Roll up, fold tiny, whatever you would have done; maybe make it into a paper airplane! Place these in an envelope. Use them in the future, or throw them across the room, and see what it feels like!

3 Writing Notes and Leaving in Random Places

Write small notes, and decorate too, if you want, they can be affirming, consoling, calming, honoring, supporting, acknowledging, approving, and/or positive. You can put these notes in tiny envelopes and write: "to whoever finds this," or just leave the notes without envelopes. When people are not watching, leave them in random places for strangers to find. These notes are gifts, random acts of written kindness, for the lucky folks who find them, and public fortune cookie messages! Maybe you will start a trend…

4 Word Quicksand

Imagine that you are writing a short letter to someone or something that will be moved by a powerful force of nature. Your letter will sink in quicksand and reach another being somewhere, it will be swept up in a tornado and land in Oz, it will be taken out to sea in a storm and land on a faraway beach, it will be burned in a wildfire and become whole again once it lands on a firefighter's hat miles away, write to a scientist on a melting iceberg in the North pole… Use your imagination and write a message that you want to send the imaginary recipient at the other end of this natural disaster. Explain in detail what this letter has gone through to reach them and where you are. Write what this disaster means to you and ask them questions about their feelings, what they have seen. Put it in an envelope and save it to read later on, maybe in a week, a month, a year…

5 Writing Releasing and the Four Elements: WRITE of passage

Write as many notes as you feel are needed about things you really need and want to let go of, release, no longer need, send away, drop, surrender, free, absolve, dissolve, or have outgrown. These can be spiritual, emotional, behavioral, relational, or anything else. Once written choose any or all of the four elements in which to create your own releasing ritual, fire, water, wind, and earth. You can carefully and safely burn, you can bury, you can let loose in the wind, you can float in liquid. Write about watching the process of transformation of these notes, where you feel this in your body, and how this ritual affected you. You might choose to do this with a witness or two, to be contained, held, supported, and loved in this WRITE of passage.

Resources

Recipes

Here is a wonderful website, PaperSlurry, on how to make handmade paper from recycled materials. You can write on your paper afterward and send the letters to people you know or don't know. Here is a link to the website:

https://paperslurry.com/blog/2014/05/19/how-to-make-handmade-paper-from-recycled-materials

Materials

Carbon copy paper is a thin blue or black piece of paper that is imbided with ink. When placed between two pieces of paper, originally in a typewriter, or written by hand, you get an exact copy of your handwriting on the bottom of the piece of paper. You can buy carbon paper online and in stationery stores. When you CC or BCC someone when sending an email, it means that you are carbon-copying them or blind carbon-copying them. Did you know that?

Seed-embedded paper is usually hand-made from recycled paper into which seeds are placed while the paper is being made. One can buy seed-embedded paper in sheets or different shapes. Once something is written on the paper it can be planted in the ground and grow surprises. You can buy seed-embedded paper online.

Movies

Mary and Max

This wonderful 2009 Claymation movie is based on a true story of a 20-year pen pal relationship between a young girl from Australia and an old man from New York. It was written and directed by Adam Elliot and produced by Melodrama Pictures in Australia.

Books

The Day the Crayons Quit by Drew Daywalt, illustrated by Oliver Jeffers.

This amazing 2013 children's book shares a series of handwritten letters composed of individual coloring crayons addressed to the young crayon owner, Duncan to communicate their complaints and frustrations with Duncan's crayon use. It was published by Philomel Books.

Places

The paper house in Rockport, Massachusetts, USA, is a house where its furniture and furnishings, including a piano, are entirely made out of rolled newspaper!

You can find out more about the house at their website: https://www.paper houserockport.com/.

Websites

The Lorelei Gruss website sells her handmade jewelry and includes Victorian Love Coins. You can learn more about it at the website: https://www.loreleigruss.com/.

MIT (Massachusetts Institute of Technology) has created a web page showing the seven different types of chain letters one can find online. You can learn more about it at on that page, appropriately titled "The seven basic types of chain letters": http://web.mit.edu/kolya/misc/txt/chain-letter-humor.

The Strangers Project's website, www.strangersproject.com, describes how the project mentioned in the chapter works.

Videos

On YouTube, you can find a brief tutorial, "How to fold a paper football," from December 6, 2008, by Fold Something, on how to fold paper into a football shape to flick a note to a classmate on the other side of the room. Here is a link: https://www.youtube.com/watch?v=a4hd1jigqLs.

References

American Antiquarian Society. (2007). *Etiquette: A history of social dance in America.* https://www.americanantiquarian.org/Exhibitions/Dance/etiquette.html

Arnold, W.N. (2004). The illness of Vincent Van Gogh. *Journal of the History of the Neurosciences, 13*(1), 22–43.

Bazelon, E., & Lennon, J.J. (2022, September 2). The prison letters project. https://www.nytimes.com/2022/09/02/magazine/prison-letters-project.html

Burgess, P. (2023). 11 of Vincent Van Gogh's most expensive paintings ever sold. *Masterworks.* https://insights.masterworks.com/art/artists/van-gogh-most-expensive-paintings/

Corrêa do Lago, P. (2018). *The magic of handwriting: The Pedro Corrêa do Lago Collection* [exhibition]. Morgan Library & Museum, New York, NY. Retrieved January 11, 2024, from https://www.themorgan.org/exhibitions/magic-of-handwriting

Dickinson, E., Johnson, T.H., & van Wagenen Ward, T. (1986). *The letters of Emily Dickinson, volume I.* Belknap Press of Harvard University Press.

Ferro, S. (2018, May 12). New museum exhibition shows off rare handwritten letters from history's most famous figures. *Mental Floss.* https://www.mentalfloss.com/article/544110/new-museum-exhibition-shows-rare-handwritten-letters-historys-most-famous-figures

Fuller Brush Company (N.D.). Retrieved January 22, 2024, from https://fuller.com/products/fuller-brush-letter-opener

Goldberg, N. (1986). *Writing down the bones: Freeing the writer within.* Shambhala; distributed by Random House.

Haynes, T. (2018, May 1). Dopamine, smartphones, and you: A battle for your time. *Harvard University the Graduate School of Arts and Sciences.* Retrieved December 23, 2023, from https://sitn.hms.harvard.edu/flash/2018/dopamine-smartphones-battle-time/

Kinsella, C., & Kaye, L. (2021, June 25). We must encourage the art of passing (virtual) secret notes in class. *Higher Education Times.* https://www.timeshighereducation.com/campus/we-must-encourage-art-passing-virtual-secret-notes-class

Lockwood, D. (2019, September 3). Anonymous stories for the Instagram age. *The New York Times.* https://www.nytimes.com/2019/09/03/arts/design/strangers-project-fountain-house-gallery.html

LoRusso, M. (2020, April 2). *How we lost the art of the signature.* The Bold Italic. https://theboldidalic.com/how-we-lost-the-art-of-the-signature-bfe63239f6b9

Love Token Society. (2012). *What are love tokens?* Retrieved December 23, 2023, from http://lovetokensociety.com/history/love-tokens/

Martin, M., & Kaur, G., (2022, December 3). What students lost since cursive writing was cut from the Common Core standards. *NPR.* https://www.npr.org/2022/12/03/1140610714/what-students-lost-since-cursive-writing-was-cut-from-the-common-core-standards

Maud, A. (2022, October 19). What is a pen pal: From then to now. *PenPal.* https://blog.penpal.me/what-is-a-pen-pal-from-then-to-now/

Murakami, H. (2000). *Norwegian wood.* Vintage International.

National Day Calendar (n.d.). *National pen pal day – June 1.* Retrieved December 19, 2023, from https://www.nationaldaycalendar.com/national-day/national-penpal-day-june-1

Stanley Gibbons (n.d.). *A guide to stamp collecting.* https://www.stanleygibbons.com/collecting-stamps/new-stamps

Steadman, C., Medway, C., & Banister, E. (2023). Consuming memorial tattoos: The body as a marketplace object? *Consumption Markets and Culture.* https://www.tandfonline.com/doi/full/10.1080/10253866.2023.2188206.

The Strangers Project. (n.d.). *What's your story?* Retrieved December 19, 2023, from https://strangersproject.com/

Van Gogh Museum. (n.d.). *5 things you need to know about Van Gogh's letters.* Retrieved December 22, 2023, from https://www.vangoghmuseum.nl/en/art-and-stories/stories/all-stories/van-goghs-letters

Varano, D. (2015, September 11). What is the history behind the unofficial USPS Motto? *USPS Blog.* https://uspsblog.com/how-is-new-york-city-related-to-famous-postal-quote/

Wire of Hope (n.d.). *Welcome to Wire of Hope's prison pen pal program.* https://wireofhope.com

Chapter 10

Caring and Restoring

Righting Ourselves Through Writing

Krystal Leah Demaine and Tamar Reva Einstein

Welcome Mat: In this chapter, caring for ourselves by using writing as a restorative gift will be explored. Lamott refers to this as unplugging, a modern way to disconnect by choice in that, "Almost everything will work again if you unplug it for a few minutes including you" (2018, p. 67). Writing communities will be addressed as will using writing to explore parts of ourselves to feel what is right for us in the moment. Writing allows us and invites us to focus on ourselves which, in this day and age, is a pregnant pause that is necessary for us to come out of the darkness of growth to the light that awaits us. Sometimes that light seems distant and at other times closer which is something to write about as well.

Restoration, Self-Care, and Writing

The word restoration can mean many things. Let's begin with that broken, cracked, antique piece of furniture you see sitting on a sidewalk. You know it has potential and you want it, but you also know that you will have to put a lot of effort into it to make it what you want it to be, right for you. You might have to strip the old paint, strengthen the foundation, change the cracked mirror, add new handles, the hinges might be rusty and need deep cleaning, and in general, this piece of abandoned, uncared-for supposed useless junk has now become, for unknown reasons, a project into which you pour enormous amounts of love, sweat, and tears.

Metaphorically, for a moment, think about the details of whatever this piece of furniture looks like in your imagination and think about yourself. When was the last time you deeply restored yourself, your spirit, your body, your psyche, your soma, your creativity, your life force, or your curiosity? As intermodal expressive arts therapists, we see beyond the brokenness, the cracks, and the peeling veneer, and imagine the process and product of artistic restoration. Soul restoration is a similar process in which we address and give care, love, and attention to things in our lives that need attention by using art, dance, music, poetry, play, drama, photography, improvisation, and, of course, all forms of self-reflective writing.

DOI: 10.4324/9781003391876-11

When we use the term restorative, we do not mean fixing, in the sense of taking your car to the garage and being able to change a part to make it run again; this is not how humans heal and that is not the message that we relate to our students. Restoration is not just about fixing; it is a whole process, and it is a life-long process. Art therapist and dream worker, Liza Hyatt, uses memoir life review writing and art responses to help others in dealing with compassion fatigue, through writing and art making and getting to what she refers to as *compassion vitality*. Hyatt (2020) says, "Writing a memoir, and making art responses to emergent themes, can empower the therapist to let go of old self-negating beliefs and behaviors and restore creative, playful vitality to both work and personal life" (p. 49).

Writing through the Best and Worst of It: What Is Hiding Under those Stumbling Stones

In hard times, we can trip over things we don't notice, our anger, our history, and our repeated self-negating behaviors, like stumbling stones. Let us stop and reflect, pause, make art, and write from these stagnant waters and move on to flowing clear streams. In the depths of boredom, sadness, anxiety, or depression, writing can invite us to give voice, expression, and validation to those feelings. In other words, we can lift ourselves out of the putrid and into beauty.

Writing has been used historically to try to make sense of our lives with and through both collective and personal traumas. Such traumas can be geopolitical, momentary, long-lasting, or ancestral, for example. The word trauma, according to Kolaitis and Olff (2017), originated from the Greek word *wound*. People have the urge to write and express their wounds, pain, challenges, and horrors that cannot be stopped. Throughout history some people have endangered themselves and their families by what they have written; there have been books burned and banned, and songs and poems have been censored, silenced, and have disappeared. Writing is not always safe, it has been done secretly in prisons, concentration camps, refugee camps, under occupation, colonialization, or slavery, during war, and in detention centers. African and African American slaves sang out loud while they were doing their forced labor, Jews and other non-Arians, who were detained by Nazis during the Holocaust, played music, put on shows, wrote poetry and stories, and painted. During occupation, Palestinians wrote and still write poetry and music, stories, and engage in many forms of art-making to express their feelings about being occupied.

Attempts to banish or weaken the arts do the opposite, and once again show us the power of the arts and writing. We are aware that we are privileged to be able to write this book and assume that those reading it are also in such a privileged state; we don't take this gift for granted. The wounds that people carry, scab over and leave both internal and external scars. These scars are often best cared for with the balm of the arts.

What follows are examples of poetry from Black American, Israeli, and Palestinian poets that are living words offering us a closer look at the emotions, in writing, of collective ancestral trauma. These poems use writing to explore collective and communal trauma, poignantly helping us understand such lived experiences. We understand that the following poets are only a very small sample of the many writers who have written about such traumas.

In the poetry of Israeli poet, Yehuda Amichai (2000), Palestinian poet, Mahmoud Darwish (2003), Arab-American poet, Naomi Shihab Nye (2002), African American poet, Langston Hughes (1995), and African American poet, Audre Lorde (2000) all address ancestral violence, trauma, grief, misplacement, displacement, fear, and longing written in visceral and powerful lines. These poets' writings are so palpable that the reader feels the trauma as they read the poet's words.

We use art and poetry-informed language to discuss trauma, instead of using trauma-informed language to discuss trauma. Instead of erasing the trauma of history, we have chosen to give honor and credence to the ancestral wounds as expressed in the poems of Israeli, Palestinian, and African American poets. Therapist and colleague to the authors, writer Nancy Scherlong, says, "Some of the best tools we have to offer trauma survivors exists in the imagination" (personal communication, November 15, 2023). The poets that we have mentioned above were blessed with the ability to transform suffering, pain, and horror through words into beautiful poems. Herein lies the gift and juxtaposition of turning to the arts in the best and worst of times. The above poetry examples allow us into a tiny part of the poet's suffering, McNiff wrote that "We become what we imagine" (1992, p. 38). In the above poems, one can only hope that the imagination is a way to get closer to what one deserves and imagines as a future emancipated human, at least one's imagination cannot be taken away, as poets have taught us. Words carry power, Jesmyn Ward (2016) has written, "I believe there is power in words, power in asserting our existence, our experience, our lives through words."

We have written poetry at the most joyous and horrific times of our lives. Writing is a way to turn over those stumbling stones. Moving the stumbling stones out of the way turns them into stepping stones on which we may step forward though their weight may always be with us.

Wholeness and Perfection: Writing from the Broken and the Whole

Life is far from perfect. We humans prefer and expect life to be smooth, a road without bumps sudden turns, or dead ends. As we have learned, the longer we live, the road of our lives is full of surprises, some welcome and some not welcome. As poet Rumi (1995) said, in the first two lines of his infamous, "The Guest House," "This being human is a guest house. Every morning a new arrival. A joy, a depression, a meanness, some momentary awareness comes as an unexpected visitor" (p. 109). The unexpected and unknown are a natural part of being alive, though often we experience these parts as extremely uncomfortable; we want a road map and we want to know who is knocking at our door.

We expect wholeness, we crave routine; for some of us, that means the routines of home life, work life, relationships, and wellness. When things break down, be they relationships or objects, when your internet slows down, your power goes out, or your car breaks down in the middle of the road, we are often surprised and very upset. Some people find these changes distressing. We don't like it when our patterns are broken.

If we look at the word broken as the opposite of whole, there are many examples that we experience during the ups and downs or the waning and waxing of our lives. Sometimes there are life events that turn us upside down that are joyous and happy but can cause us the same distress of being broken. Some of those events can include marriage, having a baby, falling in love, traveling to a new place, seeing something extremely beautiful, and creating a meaningful piece of art. There are negative and positive aspects to the changes that we as humans find difficult to digest.

During the COVID-19 lockdowns, we all experienced a collective breaking of human routine. At that time, we noticed ourselves, our communities, and even news reports and social media sharing both familiar and inventive creative acts. Our friends and colleagues wrote books, created plays, went into their music studios and recorded, among other creative acts that they often did not previously have long periods of time to work on. When there is a lack of something, food, activities, social engagement, or another resource you are used to, it can force one to call upon imagination and creativity. Some of us developed new or revisited former hobbies.

During the pandemic isolation, there was a sudden lack of flour because people had begun baking their own bread, and it was often the same people who previously had easy access to fresh baked goods whenever they wanted it. We noticed the sudden abundance of bread bakers and wondered if the lamenting of not being able to break bread with friends and families brought up this very basic food and the need for it to be made in homes. It was reported that people were making sourdough bread in particular, and, while perhaps unbeknownst to them, the fermentation in the sourdough starter can promote good digestion, and the mindful process of baking and kneading the dough can for some aid in stress reduction (Sofo, Galluzzi, Zito, 2021). When sourdough is created in the personal laboratory of one's kitchen it begins with the mixing of a starter. In Tamar's experience, a starter includes flour and water which are left in a glass jar covered with fabric, and depending on the season, the weather, or the location, the starter is fed by adding more flour or water periodically until bubbles begin to appear and there is a welcome sour aroma in the air. The process of fermentation, like the sourdough starter, can symbolize the creativity that bubbled up during the isolating times of the COVID-19 pandemic, including writing.

In another example of creativity that bubbled up during the pandemic, 380 French-speaking adult males and females, who self-identified as creative people, completed a creativity survey at the beginning of the COVID-19 lockdowns, between May and August 2020. The survey was designed to assess how creative activities might have changed without the accessibility of the community and regular routines. The participants reported that, while in lockdown, creative activities involving gardening, home arrangements, and exploring food recipes all increased. The researchers believed that the participants, since being among the creative thinking population, thrived during this time by inventing new ways to stay creatively engaged (Lopez-Persem et al., 2022). Interestingly, this thriving during a challenging and broken time, by turning to creativity, might not always be what we turn to regularly, when our routines are shattered or suddenly changed by surprise.

We also realize that making bread, revisiting hobbies, starting other new creative pursuits, or reaching out to beloveds may not have been possible during the lockdowns. The word isolation in this case takes a different turn in that there were people left alone in depression, abusive relationships, financial ruin, or lack of support services. Some people were left broken and are still in the process of repairing themselves to hopefully become whole.

In an example of feeling broken and the process of self-repairing, the writer Natalie Goldberg turned to her usual way of expression, her practice of writing, when she was told she had cancer. In an interview with for *Psychology Today*, Goldberg said, regarding her cancer diagnosis,

> But I don't mean to be flippant about cancer—it was hard, it was tough and it was scary. Then my next manuscript was about cancer because I had a whole new topic to write about. And because I wrote, it didn't take over. Writing took the chaos out of cancer
>
> (Matousek, 2016)

The brokenness of a life-endangering illness turned into a book, a story to tell aloud; Goldberg was able to put the pieces of a shattered life together by writing about the experience. The Japanese concept of *Wabi Sabi* is a wonderful metaphorical and literal practice of being attuned to the marks of imperfections and impermanence. For example, if a vessel breaks, instead of it being discarded, it is reconnected and the cracks are filled with gold as an act of remembering and honoring the breaking (Koren, 2008). Similarly, when writing about those moments when we are faced with our own imperfections, impermanence, brokenness, and the scars left in and outside is something worth exploring. Disease, wars, soul and body wounds, and natural disasters, leave marks. Do we avoid or interact with the cracks, wrinkles, scars, fading, rusting, aging, and drying up? Can we, like Goldberg, turn to writing to address, explore, and unearth what lies in our desire for perfection and wholeness; to what happens when the world around us and in us does not reveal itself as balanced, perfect, whole, or beautiful? How can the arts including writing be part of our healing process through trauma? As author and educator, Parker Palmer (2022) reminds us, "Wholeness does not mean perfection; it means embracing brokenness as an integral part of life" (p. 5).

An article in the *Harvard Business Review* reported that writing has many positive benefits for people who have experienced trauma such as reducing stress and anxiety and improving sleep. They noted that authentic writing changes a victim into a person who can now, through self-reflective writing, have ownership over the traumatic experience. Writing about or creating any art about trauma can be as painful as the trauma itself, and simultaneously creates a new story including the trauma story. "This type of immersive, reflective writing process can help us piece ourselves back together even after the most unimaginable things" (Siegel-Acevado, 2021, para 12). Trauma cannot be erased; it can be written, rewritten, and rewritten, over and over again.

Unlike Humpty Dumpty, the character in the classic children's ditty, which he cannot be put back together again after falling from a wall, it seems that we can begin to piece our parts together again, through writing and the arts. There will be signs, marks, memories, flaws, scabs, disfigurements, damages, defacements, and stains, and we might feel tainted. Our brokenness and what it leaves behind are proof that we are human and alive. Let us embrace our imperfections, though difficult, grab a pen, and begin to move it across the page. We humans yearn for wholeness.

Creative Invitations

1 **Playing with Hidden Words: Writing in Imperfect Environments**
   Sometimes, we find ourselves in places we do not want to be but know we need to be; places that are actually helping and supporting but are stressful. Writing has helped us get through these anxious moments in waiting rooms, for example. A way that Tamar uses writing in these anxious moments begins with writing a word on the top of a piece of paper and searching for all the words hidden in the word. She is very intrigued by words, by mysteries and surprises that await unconcealed. While waiting for a mammography, Tamar played with the words: mammography and mammogram. These are the words she found:

   Mom, gram, graph, rag, mam, rap, yam, fog (even though there is no 'f', spelled with a 'ph' poetic license), mama, gap, yap, my, om, am, ram, ham, or, hop, gay, may, hog, roam, ho, harp, pram, prom, and (the best for last) pray.

   Tamar was especially calmed down by the last word, "pray," and smiled. Try this hidden word in many places.
2 **Crack in the Sidewalk**

While walking look down at cracks in the sidewalk. See if the shapes, gaps, and negative spaces in the cement or stones have objects that have fallen in, been entrapped, or perhaps weeds or flowers growing in these openings. Write about the cracks in the sidewalks, and use your imagination to create stories... Maybe creatures live in them, or if you dig within you will reach an enchanted new world.

3 **Never Leave any Stone Unturned**
Go outside and turn over stones, take a photo, or draw or sculpt a visual representation of stone. What hidden treasures are there? Worms, salamanders, mud, water, moss, mushrooms? Write about finding the stone, where it is, what is under the stone, what colors and textures appealed to you about this particular stone, how big or heavy is it, what it feels like to turn it over and what this might represent in your life.

4 **Surprise in Your Pocket**
Next time you wear a piece of clothing you have not worn for a long time, put your hand in the pockets. What is there? Write about what you find; an old candy wrapper, a receipt, a note, a pair of gloves, a mushy fossilized unidentifiable object?...

5 **Torn Canvas**
Use a painting canvas that you have already begun or buy an inexpensive one at an art supply shop. Make a tiny tear with a knife anywhere on the perfect, white empty canvas. Sit in front of the canvas and write about this stage, of just making a tiny tear. Then, take your finger grab a tiny corner of the tear, and slowly rip the canvas. see what empty shape emerges. It might not feel big enough, tear a bit more. Remove the torn parts and sit again, observe the empty hole in the canvas, what shape does it evoke? Write! Then get out paints and begin painting, with the space as your guide as to what you are drawn to paint. Write at different parts of this process. Write about wholeness, damage, transformation, and the beauty of tearing.

6 **Permission Slip to Stay Home**
Use a friendly tone to write a permission slip that allows you to be late, take a day off, to not do the things that need to be done that day. Here are some examples:

- Dear Teacher: Tamar couldn't come to school today because she felt like staying in her pajamas all day.
- Dear boss: Krystal couldn't come to work today because she was better suited to curl up on the couch and read books all day long.

What are your needs and examples for your permission slips to stay home?

7 **Restoration and Care Recipe**
If you could write an ingredient list for self-care and restoration, what would be included and what would be the measurements of those ingredients? Here are some examples:

- 5 pounds of poetry books
- 1 cup of ginger tea
- A pinch of rose-scented candles
- A pint of meditation music
- A dash of cozy sweaters

8 Recipe for Eating a Book: A Metaphoric Meal for the Soul

Imagine it is lunchtime and you are very hungry. You are a creature who is nourished physically emotionally, and spiritually by ingesting books. Open your book refrigerator, look through the titles, and see which one your appetite wants that day. Pull the book out and decide: Shall I make a salad? Grill the pages? Boil them, steam them, perhaps make a sandwich? Once you have torn, cut, dissected, transformed, cooked, baked, or chopped the book up and dressed properly, begin slowly chewing. Your imaginary book-eating teeth are made for this. Savor each word, each paragraph, each chapter. Is it sweet with a happy ending? Is it sour and hard to digest, will the storyline give you heartburn? Is it a mystery and you are left asking many questions about its ingredients? Are you sated? What's for dessert? Perhaps a short poem…

9 Love Letters to the Self

Take out your most beautiful writing paper, stationery, or note paper, and begin penning a love letter to yourself. You deserve this! In fine detail tell yourself what you love about YOU. These can be physical attributes, spiritual, emotional, behavioral, or anything at all. Sign the letter and put it in an addressed envelope. Open when needed!

10 Leftover Words

Begin to save words, phrases, or sentences from auto spells, or "mistakes" you have written. Instead of discarding, deleting, or omitting these gems, revere them. Reread them through eyes of non-judgment humor, and acceptance. Enjoy the mishaps. Use them in your artmaking, your journaling, and in your own writing.

Resources

Videos

Brene Brown's TED Talk discusses her research on the *Power of Vulnerability* and has had more than 20 million views. Its success propelled her to develop trainings and write several books related to the subject. You can watch the TED talk here: https://www.ted.com/talks/brene_brown_the_power_of_vulnerability?language=en.

This documentary, "Kintsugi: Mending Memories with Gold," shows the process of Kintsugi, a part of the Japanese philosophy of wabi-sabi, the process of mending broken bowls. It was uploaded on July 9, 2023, to *On Demand* as part of their "Hometown Stories" and you can watch it here until July 9, 2025: https://www3.nhk.or.jp/nhkworld/en/ondemand/video/5003231/.

Activities

Remember the fun word template game called, Mad Libs? You can print out Mad Libs pages for FREE on this website: https://www.madlibs.com/printables/.

Places

Black Writers Museum in Philadelphia, PA, USA. There was once a time when Black Americans were not permitted to read and write. This small and mighty museum hosts workshops and exhibitions by Black American Writers. You can learn more about the museum at their website: https://www.blackwriters museum.com/.

NMAAHC Poetry Slam. The National Museum of African American History and Culture in Washington, DC, hosts an annual poetry slam each spring during National Poetry Month. Learn more about it at their website: https://nmaahc. si.edu/nmaahc-poetry-slam.

Recipes

Sourdough starter recipe. The starter is where making sourdough begins! Here is a simple recipe that we recommend trying from the King Arthur Company, found on their website:

https://www.kingarthurbaking.com/recipes/sourdough-starter-recipe.

References

Amichai, Y. (2000). *Open closed open*. C. Bloch & C. Kronfeld. (Trans.). Houghton Mifflin Harcourt.

Darwish, M. (2003). *Unfortunately, it was paradise: Selected poems*. M. Akash T & C. Forché (Trans. and Eds.). University of California Press.

Hughes, L. (1995). *The collected poems of Langston Hughes*. A. Rampersad (Ed.) and D. Roessel (Assoc. Ed.). Vintage Classics.

Hyatt, L. (2020). From compassion fatigue to vitality: Memoir with art response for self-care. *Journal of the American Art Therapy Association, 37*(1), 46–50.

Kolaitis, G., & Olff, M. (2017). Psyotraumatology in Greece. *The European Journal of Psychotraumatology, 8*(sup 4). https://doi.org/10.1080/20008198.2017.1351757

Koren, L. (2008). *Wabi-sabi for artists, designers, poets, and philosophers*. Imperfect Publishing.

Lamott, A. (2018). *Almost everything: Notes on hope*. Penguin Publishing Group.

Lopez-Persem, A., Birth, T., Quiet, S., Ovando-Telle, M., & Volle, E. (2022). Through thick and thin: Changes in creativity during the first lockdown of the COVID-19 pandemic. *Frontiers in Psychology, 13*. https://doi.org/10.3389/fpsyg.2022.821550

Lorde, A. (2000). *The collected poems of Audre Lorde*. W. W. Norton.

Matousek, M. (2016, July 19). The writing life: An interview with Natalie Goldberg. *Psychology Today*. https://www.psychologytoday.com/us/blog/ethical-wisdom/201607/the-writing-life-interview-natalie-goldberg

McNiff, S. (1992). *Art as medicine: Creating a therapy of the imagination*. Shambhala.

Nye Shihab, N. (2002). *19 Varieties of gazelle: Poems of the Middle East*. Greenwillow.

Palmer, P.J. (2022). *A hidden wholeness: The journey toward an undivided life*. Wiley.

Rumi. (1995). *The essential Rumi*. C. Barks (Trans.). Castle Books.

Siegel-Acevado, D. (2021, July 1). Writing can help us heal from trauma. *Harvard Business Review*. https://hbr.org/2021/07/writing-can-help-us-heal-from-trauma

Sofo, Galluzzi, A., & Zito, F. (2021). A modest suggestion: Baking using sourdough - a sustainable, slow-paced, traditional and beneficial remedy against stress during the COVID-19 lockdown. *Human Ecology Interdisciplinary Journal*, *49*(1), 99–105. https://www.ncbi.nlm.nih.gov/pmc/articles/PMC7880519/

Ward, J. (2016). *The fire this time: A new generation speaks about race*. Schribner.

Chapter 11

All Good Things Must Come to an End
Writing, Harvesting, and Gleaning

Krystal Leah Demaine and Tamar Reva Einstein

Welcome Mat: Writing can be likened to harvesting and gleaning in that when one writes they are collecting words that tell the stories that need to be told. As in actual agricultural harvesting, which requires hard physical work and attention to the seasons. The cyclical nature of both writing and harvesting gives us a chance to take a deeper and wider look at the writing process from beginning to end: from planting the writing seed to eating the fruits of one's labor. The blessings of what one has written are then enjoyed through gratitude and the good fortune that we writers have been gifted with can be counted word by word.

Coming to Fruition

In agriculture at the end of a growing season one harvests what one has grown. Cross-culturally, there are celebrations around the harvest season, celebrating the fruition of growth (Richardson, 2018). For example, the fall harvest is celebrated in Judaism with the holiday of Sukkot or on Thanksgiving with the harvest of the pumpkin in the United States. Many foods seasonally signal the end of a growing process that can take weeks or months. Once the fruits, vegetables, grains, legumes, and roots have been picked and stored the ground awaits replanting.

It is also important to mention that sometimes parts of the bounty are purposely left for those who are in need to glean the gifts that remain. The period in which the land lays fallow is a pause that is necessary for the future anticipated next growing season. In Judaism, every seven years farmers are asked to leave the ground fallow. This harkens back to all pauses including the Sabbath, which in Judaism is on the seventh day of the week; and from which the word sabbatical leave is derived as a pause from teaching every seven years (Eells, 1962). In some university settings, professors and faculty use their sabbaticals for writing articles and books. In arts-based academia, one might use the pause or the sabbatical for creating art, composing new music, choreographing a dance, photographing a new series, or writing a libretto.

Ironically, those who spend hours a week immersed in the teaching of creative and intellectual endeavors often do not have time to invest in their own

DOI: 10.4324/9781003391876-12

self-pollination and fertilization of their fallow fields. Therefore, as we reach the end of this writing process, we find resonance in planting, harvesting, and gleaning. We have written about transformative and restorative writing as it connects to the imagination, creative writing, journaling, self-care, metaphors, odes, hymns, prayers, childhood, children's books, the body, masks, containers, poems, libraries, notes, boxes, containers, altered books, altars, talisman, and letter writing. Our writing compass has led us through charted and uncharted waters of letters, words, sentences, paragraphs, stories, and writing processes that have reminded us of the fermentations of sourdough starters, agriculture, and the earth from stagnation to cross-pollination to compost to growing in the dark. We have also been reminded of the incomprehensible hard times that humankind has survived and is still trying to survive which has been represented in writing and through other arts. We took a walk down memory lane through our childhoods, exploring the importance of books and the continuing importance of the written word in our lives now as adults; especially, as we pass our writing and intermodal expressive art therapy experiences along to our students and clients. The seeds we have sown have come to fruition by writing this book, at least for this season.

Beauty as Healing: Altar Making and Writing

Beauty can mean many things to many people; it is a term that is multi-faceted. Like a prism, depending on where the light strikes it, there may be incredible rainbows seen on the wall, if you are paying attention, and if the sun is out! One person can be physically, spiritually, emotionally, or cognitively moved by a sunset, random acts of kindness, giving birth, caring for people at the end of their lives, hearing a piece of music for the first time, tasting something delicious, watching a footprint in the sand be taken away by a wave, recognizing a beloved by a birthmark, seeing a tree that has been turned upside down by a rain storm, finding a nest with robins' eggs in it, or being witness to a rite of passage. These are just tiny examples from a plethora of beautiful objects, people, and moments that we find beautiful in our lives. You, of course, may have many more examples of beauty and will continue to discover more; finding beauty is a process.

It is possible and probable that we do not notice beauty; we walk by beautiful objects, moments, and people without absorbing the radiant bounty of what we have just passed. Writing can help us pay attention and notice the demure and potentially overlooked gifts that the world provides us. The act of writing extrapolates and unveils the otherwise concealed experiences and stories that may be waiting for us to trip over. We feel that writing honors beauty. As we have heard many times throughout our lives, it seems, beauty really is in the eye of the beholder. Metaphorically, and literally, one can say beauty can be found everywhere and anywhere if one is aware, available, and attuned. This includes our deepest selves, our souls.

One way of honoring beauty is through altar making. In our academic and personal lives, altars are created, witnessed, and honored. Lamb (2016) says, "We make altars all the time. Some we create on purpose, some out of routine habit. The photos of your family on your hearth is an altar as such as the extensive altars inside a place of worship" (para 1). Lamb also discusses how to build an altar for transformation and intention in five steps: 1. Declare an intention, 2. Choose an altar cloth, 3. Choose meaningful symbols, 4. Bring your altar to life, 5. Work with your altar (para 5).

Tamar's small apartment is full of altars in different places and different rooms, from the living room to the bathroom. These altars are collections of objects and words that connect her, and those who visit her home, to the sacredness of the mundane, to gratitude, serenity, and kitsch and silliness. For example, her tiny bathroom is painted turquoise blue and its walls are covered in angels, made of ceramic, crochet, and other materials, that she has collected from many parts of the world. Some of the angels are on a gold-painted shelf above the toilet, including a white porcelain angel with extended wings that she brought back from a monastery in the middle of Kyiv. Angels, to Tamar, can be understood as imaginary or non-imaginary helping friends. The reason she keeps them in the bathroom is that she believes that bodily acts are something that we do not often pay attention to until our bodies begin to malfunction. These angels are in the bathroom to remind Tamar to stay grateful that her body is working properly.

In other parts of Tamar's house, in different corners and niches, one can find smaller altars as reminders of beloveds who are no longer here in person. In addition, there are multi-cultural symbols juxtaposed together in an act for a wish for peace. On a shelf in Tamar's kitchen, where she lights her Jewish Shabbat candles, there are also two Buddha candle holders, one antique brass Islamic container with its candle lit on the inside with text from the Koran on the outside, and two tall glass guardian angel Christian candles bought at a Botanica in New York City. Another notable altar that Tamar has in her apartment is the one dedicated only to incense burning, and most of the altars include the five-fingered *hamsa* symbol, the hand of Fatima, and blue and white evil eyes which are all symbols of protection.

Krystal is highly attuned to the presence of objects and spaces that, to her, are altars almost everywhere she goes. For example, when walking out of an asphalt parking lot she looked down trying to remember if she had taken everything she needed to teach that day, and was stunned by a stone sparkling in the sun, sitting on a dried-out leaf, to Krystal this is an altar of nature. She might then pick it up and put it on her desk for the day, then return it to the parking lot later, to remind her of the sacred beauty that is all around us. Some altars are impermanent, especially in nature. For example, Krystal's son kicked snow while walking to the car and a heart of snow landed at Krystal's feet. Although we know that heart-shaped snow will melt, for that moment, the heart became an altar that Krystal will photograph to save. Perhaps Krystal will add that photograph to the next altar she makes at home.

Altar finding and creating is available and attainable anywhere; be it in Krystal's classroom, her car, her office, outdoors, or various spaces in her home. The altar is placed in a location where Krystal is invited to be reminded to pause, reflect, and ponder the intentions, wishes, hopes, and sometimes prayers that the combination of the objects brings forth. Her altars have included objects such as mementos from childhood, photographs, nature elements, things that bring light such as candles and crystals, and scents including oils and sticks of incense. A particularly important altar in Krystal's home is the one she created in honor of her father when he passed away. This altar is placed in the central part of her home, a small cupboard-filled room adjacent to the kitchen pantry, which was once referred to as the "butler's pantry" (Primavera, 2023) that slowly and organically became a sacred place that she walks through each day. The objects in Krystal's altar stay the same except for the Jewish memorial *yahrzeit* candle which is lit at different meaningful and important times of the year. Walking by her father's altar every day on the way to cutting vegetables in the kitchen gives her a chance to pause and remember her dad; a way of slowing down as she moves quickly through many nurturing and nourishing daily activities in her life.

While some altars in Krystal's life may stay in the same location for a long time, her classroom altars are removed by the end of the meeting that day. Varying in size, material, and location, the classroom altar is important in that it allows a personal spiritual, calming, and grounding presence for Krystal. Altars in the classroom send a signal that this is a special place and something different is about to happen here. In Krystal's classroom, she places objects in the middle of the room, on a piece of fabric, which serves as an altar; it is a meditation or grounding place and also invites the prompt for the day. Krystal has used the same piece of multi-colored fabric for the last 21 years since she has been teaching undergraduate students. Altars in academic settings are very different from personal altars at home. In the classroom, Krystal places objects in the middle of the room to spark a story, a narrative, an interplay of words; begin a discussion; or open the topic for the day. Sitting in a circle around this altar, which symbolizes a non-traditional way of sitting in a classroom, can invite a few moments of writing, sketching, or playing a quiet musical instrument as the students prepare for the learning that is to come.

Each of our personal altars might seem very different, but actually they are deeply connected in that they evoke contemplation, connection, protection, memories, and a sense of grounding and rooting. We acknowledge and are grateful for those who came before us and for the experiences that have built us, and that will continue to help us grow through these altars.

Pausing: Stop and Smell the Stories

Writing is an invitation to pause, to pay attention, to see, to listen, to feel, to taste; in essence, the act of writing is a way to stop ourselves in our tracks and sit and release through the penned words that flow from us. Writing, like reading, can transport us to other realms, to move through time and place, while sitting still. This is the magic of writing. By stopping, we move inwards, then outwards. By pausing, we invite ourselves to discover what may have been hidden from us before the pause.

According to the Lurianic Kabbalistic creation story, when God created light there was so much of it that it had to be put in vessels (Drob, 2023). The light was so powerful that even the vessels that God created could not contain the intense light. The glass vessels shattered and the light was dispersed throughout the world and hidden in all of the corners and crevices all over the globe and are still there for all humans to find. For us, it seems very important, especially in the darkest of times, that we can hope to find a glimmer of light hidden in a crevice somewhere, even inside ourselves, and then write about it.

Pausing is also experienced differently at different stages of our lives. In the children's book *Wait* by Antionette Portis (2015), an adult is rushing a child along with her to catch the train. The child repeatedly asks the grownup to wait, to which the response is to hurry. The adult is focused on one thing, to be on time for the train, while ignoring the child's curiosity and desire to share with the adult the wonderful things the child is seeing and discovering along the way. In this story, beauty is seen by the child and finally at the end of the book, realized by the adult. We see this simply written story as a wonderful example for adults. Often when we rush to a destination, we can become blind to our surroundings and the beauty they hold.

Learning to slow down is at the core of Buddhist teachings. The overwhelming demands and high expectations of the modern world can take a toll on us. Eastern traditions and rituals explore practices to help us live through and with modern-day demands. Thích Nhất Hạnh's book titled *No Mud No Lotus* (2014) refers to the Buddhist concept of acknowledging suffering as we experience beauty; we can't expect a life without suffering and we can't expect beauty without life, they go hand in hand. Hạnh says, "We must remember that suffering is a kind of mud that we need to generate joy and happiness" (p. 13). Therefore, the title of Hạnh's book, *No Mud No Lotus*, refers to how the lotus needs to grow through the mud, or in our language, how suffering can be a fertile place in which to grow through the arts and writing. Through practice: different forms of meditation, mindfulness, sitting quietly, calligraphy, painting, sculpting, embroidering, knitting, mandala making, writing, or making altars; one sits in the metaphorical mud and then sees the miraculous growth of the lotus. The beautiful lotus flower blooms out of the ooziness of mud. In other words, there are exquisite, enchanting, and dazzling gems awaiting you in the darkest corners to write about, they are hidden in the mud. You might have to sit in the dark to find the jewels of your story. As attributed to Dr. Martin Luther King Jr. (1968) among others, "Only when it is dark enough can you see the stars" (para 7).

Writing offers a pause to focus on the present moment. As we discussed in Chapter 4, it is paying attention to details that slow the writer down to notice the minute or seemingly mundane. A pause for details helps us distill what we are writing into a deeper, richer, and more flavorful cauldron of words, sentences, and stories. Mindful writing brings us to a sensory level, noticing the movement of the pen, the interplay of light, and the focus on just doing one thing: writing! Our descriptive writing allows us to see what we are writing about, to taste it, and to bring it to life. You might consider meditation as a practice of complete stillness; however, the choreography of our hand moving a pen across a page in a repetitive dance of words is a form of mindfulness, a practice of presence, and an act of meditation.

The Rubin Museum website (2018) discusses the process of engaging with art as a meditation. It is suggested that looking at the details of the art, contemplating the art, and focusing on the art becomes a mindful practice of presence; and the act of mindful meditation begs us to stay present in the moment (The Rubin, 2018). Along these lines, the same could be said for engaging in music-making, painting, dance, or writing. As Biswas (2011) wrote, there is a similar physiological engagement in music-making as there is in meditation; suggesting a relationship between breath in music and meditation practice, as well as the focus of attention, and the shift in consciousness; in this case perhaps it is the moment of flow that takes over when we make music or when we meditate. In relationship to reading and writing, Moffett (1983) considers both as a form of meditation, in the way that the engagement allows one to focus on their "inner stream of consciousness" (p. 315).

On a personal level, for Krystal who maintains a strong mindful practice, music-making practice, and writing practice, the parallel is crystal clear. She has noticed an overlapping sense of rhythm, whole bodily calming, and emotional excitement in her engagement with these forms; furthermore, there is an evocation, and a desire to ponder and reflect after each act. Also, Krystal feels the interweaving of all of the colors of each part of this practice once she sits up and faces the day and might take a protective and nurturing shawl, blanket, or talisman with her as a reminder of inner quiet and groundedness. As emphasized by Tara Brach (2023),

> Through the sacred art of pausing, we develop the capacity to stop hiding, to stop running away from our experience. We begin to trust in our natural intelligence, in our naturally wise heart, in our capacity to open to whatever arises.
>
> (p. 50)

Many cultures, traditions, religions, spiritual communities, and individuals practice the importance of taking a pause; through prayer, chanting, yoga, Tai Chi, Qi Gong, meditation, writing, and other arts (Mani, 2018). Some traditions overlap, and some are similar or might remind us of other rituals, of taking time out to recalibrate, to stop our habitual behaviors and daily routines. Some folks go on retreats to deepen their practices and to learn how to become more immersed in calming rituals within their busy daily lives. We might have been taught that resting, pausing, napping, or taking breaks are signs of weakness, of not keeping up with the rhythm expected from us; that our "lagging," does not fit in. We want to remember how poignantly Thoreau (1910) wrote, "If a man does not keep pace with his companions, perhaps it is because he hears a different drummer. Let him step to the music which he hears, however measured or far away" (p. 430). Most of us do not have the luxury in our modern, western lives to completely remove ourselves and move into the forest and live in a cabin, meditate on nature, and write about it, as Thoreau did. We do, however, have the capability and ability to internalize the experience by engaging in activities that connect us to deep inner and outer quiet, to the sacredness of nature, to writing, art making, and to the outer and inner seasons within us all.

In this busy world, where children are pulling their parents by the hand to stop and taste, see, and smell the stories they are rushing by, perhaps we can begin to slow down, step by step, to allow ourselves to notice, and absorb what is around us; to stop and smell the stories.

Creating Community with Writing: Weaving a Word-Based Kinship

Writing is often considered a lonely art form. One may sit in a room alone for hours a day writing in solitude. To write, many people need a very quiet atmosphere. Although, as we previously discussed in Chapter 2, there are writers whose writing thrives in a public environment, perhaps surrounded by strangers, sounds, and maybe the smell of coffee. Krystal loves writing in the public environment, the more sounds, people, scents, and disruptions, the better she writes, and it keeps her on her writing toes! And ironically, while we crave this silent space for writing we also need witnessing, listening, and containing for what we have written.

There are writers, Tamar being one of them, who write well in online community writing groups, as do her group mates who have become a chosen family that shares intimate writing. Co-writing this book, was also an experience of writing in community through a dyad. Originally, we thought we would each write one chapter and send it to one another, but we discovered quickly that we needed to write this book together by meeting online weekly which became daily. Spending hours of writing together, live, online, conversing, laughing, crying, and enjoying the experience thousands of miles apart.

McNiff (2003) suggested that there is a special kind of energy that is manifested by creating in collaboration with groups. In tune with this suggestion, Ridley, Einstein, and McNutt (2023) described their collaborative online art-based community which was born during the COVID-19 pandemic and continues until today; writing about the process was restorative and affirming.

In Krystal's foundations of expressive therapies course, she introduces creative and expressive writing and community to her undergraduate students by laying a diverse collection of international postcards which she has collected for over many years. Over 100 postcards are placed face-up on top of the tapestry in the middle of the room. Her students surround the fabric sitting on the floor in a circle. The images on the cards include colorful doors in Dublin, Hokusai's "Great Wave off Kanagawa," and Salvador Dali's "The Elephants" for example. All of the images are appreciated for their cultural roots and diversity.

Krystal asks her students to take a few moments to look at the images on the cards, choose one that they resonate with, and bring that one card back to their seats. She then gives the students three minutes to draw a quick sketch of the image on the card in their journal and reminds them that the heart of the task is about writing, and the drawing simply is to offer a visual representation, a reminder of the forms and shapes seen on the card that they chose. After the students draw their brisk illustration, they are asked to write a list of every color, shape, form, and object that they observe on the card. She then asks the students to write the mood and emotions they feel when looking at the card, as well as associations: the year, season, day, location, and the time they believe the image was set. Next, Krystal gives the students ten minutes to look at the card and write the story they see using the words that they have written. Any other ideas, feelings, images, and resonances are welcome in their writing.

After the students are finished writing for ten minutes Krystal asks them to turn to the people near them and to make a group of four. Each person in the small group is asked to show the postcard image and read the story that they wrote, meanwhile, the three other students are asked to listen deeply and collaboratively determine one phrase that encapsulates the reader's postcard image. Once the phrase or sentence is determined, it is written down on a blank strip of paper that Krystal handed out to each student earlier. At the end of the small group readings, each student has a phrase to go along with their postcard. The students are told that their cards will become part of a larger community story. They are asked to hold onto their strip of paper with the phrase, then they place their postcards in a large half-circle arc on the fabric. Once they have witnessed and looked deeply at the placement of their card in what has become a story arc, Krystal asks them to move their image cards in an order that allows the story to make sense to them both personally and as a group. As the story begins, they are asked to pay attention to the beginning, middle, and end. All stories have a beginning, middle, and end. Once the image story has been created, and agreed upon by all, the phrases are placed underneath each corresponding image card. Krystal asks the group to cover or close their eyes while sitting in their seat, and simply listen while she reads the phrases aloud that have now become their communal shared story. After the first reading and listening, the students are often astonished by the natural flow and magical connections of the phrases read together that have become an organic story. Until you are an active participant in an image-based and word-based group experience similar to the postcard-phrase-story exploration, you may find it hard to believe that personal associations, feelings, and ideas are so interwoven. There is a synchronicity that happens in these moments that is often unexplainable but felt.

Creative Communities: COVID Isolation Sparking the Imagination

Born out of the COVID-19 pandemic, when we were not allowed to gather in groups, the Listening Hour, an idea conceptualized by Jonathan Fox, allowed people to meet online in a small group with a facilitator for one hour of shared group storytelling. Fox was the innovator behind Playback Theater, a method he developed in 1975 that involves listening to a story told by an audience member which is subsequently performed by an acting troupe before the audience (Listening Hour, 2020). Krystal participated in a Listening Hour group during the first year of the pandemic. She shared a memory from her childhood which exemplified her relationship with her sisters at the time. The process struck a chord with her in feeling connected to the strangers with whom she was sharing her story and she was so moved by the power of their silent, active, online listening and witnessing that she became tearful yet also felt happy to be heard. Indeed, Krystal was so moved by the experience that six months later she completed the Listening Hour training, and became a Listening Hour certified practitioner. Krystal finds it essential for her growth as a Listening Hour practitioner to take notes and write a reflection on her experience after she facilitates a session.

During the pandemic isolation, academic instruction, was moved to an online platform. For us, as educators, we noticed that moving online caused a sudden separation and disconnection; meeting in person was severed and all of a sudden, the instructors and students were people in little black boxes on computer screens. Teaching expressive arts therapy is immersive, hands-on, and experiential, requiring physical and social interaction, witnessing of emotion, and attunement with others. All those who were teaching online had to find novel ways to keep their students engaged while maintaining the integrity of their instruction. As the semester progressed and the unknown was just as present and frightening as it was from the start, we noticed that our students, participants, and colleagues began to feel very helpless.

While planning for her online graduate course, Tamar decided to create a group arts-based and writing exploration to address this feeling of living in limbo, in a constant state of the unknown. Tamar invited each student within a wonderfully culturally rich combination of women, Jews, Arabs, religious, secular, homosexual, and heterosexual students to imagine a female character from a childhood book or film that they saw as a heroine. Tamar and the students listened to the names and stories of these strong, magical, powerful, female characters. Some were from ancient fairy tales, others from films, and some from books the students' grandparents had brought from foreign lands.

Tamar then asked the students to draw, paint, or sketch the heroine that they chose. In the next class, the students and Tamar viewed and witnessed the art online together and discussed how they related to the art as humans related to the characters, to the interweaving, juxtapositions, and connections. Some of the strong female heroines that the students chose to invoke, conjure, and illustrate in their drawings included Pippi Longstocking, Ursula from *The Little Mermaid*, Mary Poppins, and many other wonderful women and girls. The students then wrote lists of words about what they saw, felt, imagined, and associated with every character; in addition to the magical powers they needed from each of those female characters, at the time of the pandemic.

The lists the students wrote were combined into a group fairy tale, which started very organically. One student volunteered to be a scribe. The other students took turns and sometimes spoke over each other excitedly, as they created sentences from the strengths of the characters. These sentences turned into paragraphs which then turned into a whole new fairy tale. The tale was affirming, humorous, serious, beautiful, and full of female power. The new story created a community of women from many walks of life who were all reminded that their group superpowers could be even stronger when held and contained in the communal new narrative; a way for the women to affirm their own superpowers. Some said that they couldn't wait to tell this story to their own children, that they felt closer to each other now, and that the entire experience reminded them of their inner strengths during uncertainty and upheaval. We remember fairytales as stories that include journeys on which there were protective characters, magical powers, and frightening or traumatic challenges. Fairytales can be a wonderful genre of writing for self-reflection, education, and therapy touching on the emotions of joy, suffering, danger, and freedom.

Tamar discovered early in the pandemic that she craved writing communities after many years of writing alone. Tamar never really paid attention to how important writing was to her—until during the COVID-19 lockdowns when she signed up for online writing groups. She looked up to writers like Oliver Sacks and Irving Yalom who, in her eyes, page by page told stories about their work as healers in a humane, personal, and accessible manner and style. These authors' authenticity moved her. She searched for writing groups that were soul-based and could allow for intimate writing. Surprisingly, now, a few years later, not only did she find new shared writing homes, but also writing friendships, tribes, families, and solid communities steeped in words and love. Specifically, the spiritual poetry class at *Tiferet Journal* has become a place where Tamar can write share, and listen to poetry that distills emotions, current events, and people's life stories that get to the essence of it all.

In Levine's book *Poesis* (1997), he reminds the reader that presence is a gift in itself, a present through presence. When expressive arts therapy students present their own suffering, pain, and joy and all of their life experiences authentically through the arts, in a group, and then are given feedback in the same manner, the outcome of this gift exchange is the table on which the feast will be set. Levine refers to the "feast" as a soul and arts-based meal, made of both the person giving the art and the offering of arts-based feedback given by the group. Community is the basis of this work; there needs to be a presenter and receivers, a group that receives the gift. The process of bearing gifts to the feast (Levine, 1997) is about the ritual of presentation; this ritual brings up associations to the authors of being invited to a feast of intermodal expressive arts therapy and writing delicacies. Bon Appetit!

In our classes, at the end of the semester, when things are coming to a close, we both create a ritual of sharing and gift exchange as we have learned and experienced from many of our beloved mentors through their workshops, classes, and books (Knill, Barba, Fuchs, 2005; Levine,1997; McNiff, 1998). Outside of our roles as teachers, we are both aware as people who have worked in end-of-life care, that discussing endings and saying goodbye can be challenging to explore and create, and are often avoided. In our academic roles, we feel that it is our responsibility to model the inclusion of arts-based rituals and teach ways of parting from one another. The rituals and the exchanges that we call upon are always steeped in the arts and writing. When a course comes to an end, like the transition between seasons, there is harvesting to be done. We have been fortunate to have studied and gleaned wisdom and experience from intermodal expressive arts-rooted teachers and founders. Our writing this book, in a sense, is a harvesting of many years of fruitful work.

Creative Invitations

1 **Superheroes**

Think about characters in books that you have read, either as a child or an adult that inspired you and made you feel that you wish you had some of their powers, strengths, or talents. Choose one character. Write a list of the words that describe that character. Take those words and write a short poem adding as many other words as you need and dedicate it to yourself. You might even want to use your own name instead of the characters' names. Read out loud and see how it feels to own what the character owned. If the muse befalls you, draw an illustration to accompany this poem. Try this invitation as much as you would like with different characters.

2 **Finding Beauty**

Take a photograph of a moment of beauty that you accidentally discover. Sit in front of the photograph and carefully look at all the tiniest details in the image. If you are looking at your phone you can zoom into certain parts, if the photo is printed you can look at the details with a magnifying glass. Write a short story about where you took the photograph, the time of day, your mood when you took it, your mood now, and what this moment of beauty added to your life. Repeat when necessary. You might find that this will become a practice regularly.

3 Creating Your Altar

Find a space in your home that feels right for your altar. The space might be public, such as the living room, or private in a closet on a shelf. Think about what is inviting you to create this altar and connect objects that are connected to your feelings and imaginings of how this altar will serve you. Once you have collected the objects, take time to place them in a way and on a surface that feels right to you. Walk away, leave it alone, and then come back and see if there is something you feel you want to add or take away. If altar-making becomes part of your life, continue this process in other parts of your home. You might create rituals around these altars in your home. We would like to invite you to use the written word as part of your altar, either in small notes, letter writing, post-its, or any other form of words; carved into clay or stone, cutouts from magazines, or words from books that you find inspiring.

Resources

Movies

Disney's animated film *Coco* shows a wonderful example of a Mexican altar offering food and drink to ancestors.

Writers Groups

One of the ways to become a stronger writer is by joining a writer's group. Below are some places that often offer writing classes

- Abbey of the Arts, among other things, offers seasonal writing groups that are often connected to the Celtic Calendar, taught by Christine Valter Painter. Find out more here:
  https://abbyofthearts.com.
- Tiferet Journal offers spiritual poetry writing courses taught by Donna Baier Stein. Find out more here: https://tiferetjournal.com/.
- Upaya Zen Center offers contemplative Zen-based writing classes, some poetry and haiku, and sometimes taught by Natalie Goldberg. Find out more here: https://www.upaya.org.

References

Biswas, A. (2011). The music of what happens: Mind, meditation, and music as movement. In D. Clarke & E. Clarke (Eds.), *Music and consciousness: Philosophical, psychological, and cultural perspectives*. (pp. 95–110). Oxford University Press.

Brach, T. (2023). *Radical acceptance: Embracing your life with the heart of a Buddha.* Bantam Books.

Drob, S. (2023). *Kabbalistic visions: C.G. Jung and Jewish mysticism* (2nd ed.). Routledge.

Eells, W.C. (1962). The origin and early history of sabbatical leave. *American Association of University Professors, 48*(3), 253–256.

Hạnh, T.N. (2014). *No mud no lotus.* Parallax Press.

King, M.L., Jr. (1968, April 3). "I've been to the mountaintop" [speech]. Mason Temple, Memphis, TN. https://www.afscme.org/about/history/mlk/mountaintop

Lamb, L. (2016, February 23). Building altars for personal transformation. *Spirituality+Health.* https://www.spiritualityhealth.com/articles/2016/02/23/building-altars-personal-transformation

Levine, S.K. (1997). Bearing gifts to the feast: The presentation as a rite of passage in the education of expressive therapists. In S.K. Levine (Ed.), *Poiesis: The language of psychology and the speech of the soul* (pp. 43–61). Jessica Kingsley Publishers.

Listening Hour. (2020). *Home.* https://www.listeninghour.org/

Mani, L. (2018). *Sacred secular: Contemplative cultural critique.* Routledge.

McNiff, S. (1998). *Trust the process: An artist's guide to letting go.* Shambhala.

McNiff, S. (2003). *Creating with others: The practice of imagination in life, art, and in the workplace.* Shambhala.

Moffett, J. (1983). Reading and writing as meditation. *Language Arts, 60*(3), 315–322.

Portis, A. (2015). *Wait.* Roaring Brook Press.

Primavera, B. (2023, May 9). The evolution of the kitchen pantry through the centuries. *The Examiner News.* https://www.theexaminernews.com/the-evolution-of-the-kitchen-pantry-through-the-centuries/

Richardson, B. (2018). *Thanksgiving & other festivals of the harvest.* Mason Crest.

Ridley, S., Einstein, T., & McNutt, J. (2023). Exploring making art in community through zoom during the COVID-19 pandemic. *Journal of Applied Arts & Health, 14*(2), 1–13. https://doi.org/10.1386/jaah_00137_1

The Rubin. (2018, August 31). *Art as meditation: A lesson in mindfulness.* Retrieved January 3, 2024, from https://rubinmuseum.org/art-as-meditation-a-lesson-in-mindfulness

Thoreau, H.D. (1910). *Walden.* Thomas Y. Crowell & Company.

Chapter 12

Leftovers
Gleaning from the Scribbles in the Margins

Krystal Leah Demaine and Tamar Reva Einstein

Welcome Mat: Gleanings are the leftovers at the end of a harvest; what is reaped by those who look and find what the harvesters have left. We liken these gleanings to those writings in the margins; to words, sentences, and sketches, those sometimes impossible to read scribbles we penned. These leftovers are filled with nutrients for the soul, mind, and spirit. This chapter addresses those written remnants.

The Gleanings

Sometimes what we write in the margins of our notebooks and books is more interesting than the text. As the choreographer, dancer, and writer, Twyla Tharp (2003) remarked, "Everything is raw material. Everything is relevant. Everything is usable. Everything feeds into my creativity" (p. 10). Those legal pads with large empty spaces to the left of the lines are such wonderful places to scribble and sketch; mindlessly. Our writing in the margins can be useful. Do you ever write in the margins of the books that you read, the notes that emerge from your stream of consciousness? Have you ever found other people's writings in the margins of the books that you borrowed from the library or perhaps purchased at a used bookshop? Those notes that you write in the margin can perhaps be the most important part of what the book means to you, perhaps the notes are what you have gleaned from the reading. Those important thoughts, feelings, and imaginings, came up and were evoked by the words that were written by the author of that book. When we write in the margins of a legal pad, for example in a class, when we are taking notes, it might be interesting to go back and look at only what was written in the margins, to see where our unconscious went while our brain was consciously focused on the class itself.

As we wrote, revised, wrote some more, and finally edited this book, we were left with a smorgasbord of leftovers. We want to give recognition to some of the leftovers and gleanings.

We have written this book from our own experiences. We realize that others have different experiences with writing. We have no intention of harming

DOI: 10.4324/9781003391876-13

others or misconstruing history. In our own lives, we strive and work hard to be aware, honor, and appreciate cultural, racial, and all human sameness and differences. Writing freely is not to be taken for granted, there are many places in the world where people are not able to write freely. We hope that this book gives readers a comfortable invitation to write from emotional places and geo-political spaces.

Playing with Writing: Taking Ourselves Less Seriously Word by Word

An area that we wish we could have given more attention to is playfulness in writing. The importance of playful writing as adults is an important part of self-care. This is different from how we discussed playing with words as children in Chapter 6; remember the imaginary food, "pepolish?" We are referring to the innate need to be silly at any age which is often looked down upon in adult society. Silliness is a way of paying attention to the parts of us that are tired of being responsible adults 24/7. We are allowed to let go of grown-up behaviors by being improvisational in a natural way through all of the arts including writing. This is what makes engaging in the arts such a sacred act. Playfulness and the arts are the only places where adults get to act out their deepest emotions and play with them. We have personally and professionally witnessed and experienced a lot of ripping paper, breaking things, running around, playing drums loudly, storytelling, dancing, getting paint all over our hands, crying, laughing, yelling, writing, and communicating anything that needs to be expressed; all forms of grown-up play. Continual playing for as long as we live, in whatever art form or craft one uses, is a way of keeping the imagination and creativity from becoming rusty, as we mentioned earlier; we believe play to be the preventative balm for our souls and spirits. Playing is serious in the arts, silliness is no-nonsense for adults, so play and be silly when you create and grow. We know that not every cloud has a silver lining and that one can explore all of the paradoxes of clouds and humans through writing and the arts, whatever lining your cloud might have. We know from our own lives that the silver linings are not always visible or available to us when everything is dark, cloudy, sad, and we do not see the light at the end of the tunnel. We gently suggest using writing and all of the arts, though it might feel impossible to create anything when we are enveloped by such dark clouds. Let's not forget that the dark clouds finally begin to shed their tears releasing what has been held inside of them.

We want to give tribute to other ways we have used letters, words, and writing for play in childhood and adulthood. You might recognize some of these letter games and word games and you may not. According to *The Paris Review* (Raphel, 2020), word games, like some of the following, weren't recorded as official games until 1913. However, we imagine that similar games may have been enjoyed by people of all ages preceding that date by thousands of years. We have taken the artistic license to add spelling bees, riddles, tongue twisters, and limericks as word games. Here is our list of some word games:

- Scrabble®
- Mad Libs®
- Bananagrams®
- Boggle®
- Wordle®
- Story Cubes®
- tongue twisters
- limericks
- crossword puzzles
- Scattergories®
- spelling bee
- riddles
- Hangman

You may have other word games to add to this list depending on where and when you grow up. If so, please write about those games in your journal and teach the games to those around you to keep them going. We would also like to share childhood memories of playing with words through food. As we mentioned in Chapter 2, as children we were told not to play with our food; and we suggested that we play with words as we played with food, as if you were an infant, in your high chair, tasting, mushing, and playing with food for the very first time. We had a sudden revelation from our childhood that we had forgotten an important way of playing with words and letters: AlphaBits® and alphabet soup, a break-fast cereal, and a hot soup, in which the letters were part of what you ate. We enjoyed moving the letters around in the milk or the soup and creating words with the letters we found. Once we were happy with the words, we had created with our noodle or cereal letters, we ate our words.

We love words! We realize that there are words that we repeated in this book and some that just didn't make it in, but we love them all, we just can't have them all. Instead of this, we've made a list, almost like one makes a shopping list, of words that we want to use in future writings. We are not sure what shop to buy these in, we have not yet found an official word shop; meanwhile, we have made an official wish list, and hope to find a proper home for these words in the future.

garish, lavish, subtletude, minuet, impetus, eschew, dabble, obliterate, plentitude, spectacle, acumen, insidious, proclivity, candor, sunset, burgeon, proliferate, perforate, misty, affectionate, tenuous, impervious, menagerie, coalesce, pious, iridescent, ameliorate, clairvoyant, chancellor, amorphous, bosom, sponge cake, burgeoning, dandy, stupendous, bungalow, aubergine, argyle, Madagascar, surely, whippersnapper, cottage, labyrinth, sequoia, ladybug, strawberry, cantaloupe, arabesque, amethyst, cardamom, effervescent, epsilon, rapture, equanimity, forerunner, fungus, camembert cheese, bumble, artichoke, chameleon, jaunt, leisure, gargantuan, tarantula, polarity, counterpoint, pistachio, askew, refrain, bisque, chrysanthemum, sprightly, slinky, serendipitous, unabashed, determinism, accentuate, luscious, opalescence…

This is only a small shopping list of words. We look forward to contributing more to this list in the future, but for now, all good things must come to an end.

Creative Invitations

1 **Lists of Words You Love**
   Imagine a store that is stocked with words on the shelves all placed in alphabetical order. Some of the words are in bags, some in boxes, some need to be weighed, and some of them edible and others not. As you roam this word market, fill your shopping cart with your most beloved words. You can get more than one word that you love if you so choose. For example, if you want to add ten pounds of "love" or three kilograms of "magic," you may add them to your cart. After checking out, take your words home, and use them in any way you choose. For example, write with them, build an altar out of them, make a collage with them, write a song with them, hang them up on wind chimes or as a mobile, or put them in envelopes and send them to people you love.

2 **Leftovers that Have to Do with Meals**
   While you are preparing a meal, take pictures of the piles of leftover raw ingredients that you are cooking with; the onion skins, the carrot peels, the coffee grinds, and the lemon seeds. Take pictures of these piles, this amazing colorful nest, at all different angles. After you put your food in the stove or the oven, look at the photographs and think about these leftovers. Write the associative words that come to you from the photographs of the piles of leftovers you did not use in your cooking; the colors, the textures, the scents, the shadows, the light, the potential, who might enjoy them: animals, insects, a compost pile? After you write the associative words go check on your food to make sure it is not burning, then go back to your words and see if you can write a short story about where these leftovers would like to be, what they would like to become, or who they would like to feed.

3 **Fast forward/part II**
   After the meal has been eaten by you and/or your guests, you have done the dishes, and your guests have left, turn off most of the lights, except for one light shining in the kitchen. Take photos of the glasses, soup bowls, pots, and pans, and contemplate what the clean dishes remind you of, what was in

them, and what has occurred. Remember the aftermath. The meal comes to an end but food is served in them and those containers all have stories to tell. Write down what the soup bowls have to disclose, what the glasses have to share, and what tale the forks have to spin.

4 **List of Silly, Non-Sense, Gibberish, and Pig-Latin Words**

Close your eyes and try hard to think back to the last time you wrote or spoke a silly non-sense gibberish or pig-Latin word. You may be surprised that you wrote a silly or non-sense word today on your phone because of auto-correct. We tend to delete our automatically corrected misspelled words, however, you might consider saving them because they can be used for future reference. Be as ludicrous as possible, use as much poppycock as you desire, allow malarky to guide you, blabber, and be as foolish and senseless as possible as you write these words! Once you have written your list of words and your memory has been refreshed to all of the words that you hardly ever use, that have been stored away in your repository of word hogwash, remove those words and honor them, write with them; the silly words deserve your attention, especially if they make you laugh!

Resources

Articles

Did you know that you can regrow fresh vegetables the leftover scraps? You could grow fresh leeks from the leftover bulb-like stalks, or celery from their leafy heads. The 2018 *Garden Tech* article by Jolene Hansen titled "How to Grow Vegetables from Table Scraps" will help you learn more. You can also search for videos and other written resources on how to grow vegetables from scraps. Here is a link to the Hansen article: https://www.gardentech.com/blog/gardening-and-healthy-living/growing-food-from-kitchen-scraps.

The article, *An Artist's* Blue, published in the Deccan Herald discusses Yves Klein who died young, at 34. His art and performances were unforgettable and highly unusual. Yves was an artist who made art through challenges and was unwilling to bend to societal norms of the art of his time. He left behind some important leftovers for artists to come.

Here is a link to the Yves Klein article: https://www.deccanherald.com/features/an-artists-blue-2048726

Book

The Diving Bell and the Butterfly (2008) by Jean-Dominique Bauby (Knopf).

This book is a memoir of a man who was surprised by a sudden fatal illness, in his 40s. His book was written, as he died, with the blinking of his eyes, letter by letter, word by word. An incredible leftover for all writers and readers. Writing has no limits it seems!

As Baby wrote, "once, I was a master of recycling leftovers. Now I cultivate the art of simmering memories." (Bauby, 2008, p. 36).

References

Raphel, A. (2020, March 23). A brief history of word games. *The Paris Review*. https://www.theparisreview.org/blog/2020/03/23/a-brief-history-of-word-games/

Twyla Tharp, Mark Reiter (2003). *The creative habit: Learn it and use it for life*. Simon and Schuster.

After-Words

A Thank-You Note to the Book

Krystal Leah Demaine and Tamar Reva Einstein

Dear Book,

We have reached the end of a process together, the three of us, Tamar, Krystal, and you, dear book! We are grateful that we have been given the gift of writing, thinking, erasing, imagining, sharing, laughing a lot, complaining, editing both your pages and our thoughts, emoting, researching, reading, drinking lots of tea, and working together, with a seven-hour time difference.

At the end of this path, we appreciate writing even more than when we began. We have learned some interesting and juicy tidbits. We have thought deeply about how writing colors our teaching habits, and how our writing habits color us. All of the arts, your first cousins, our beloved book, have been mentioned and revered alongside your expressive, therapeutic, nurturing, transforming, restorative, and guiding powers word by word.

As a metaphor for trees, in a body where physical books begin, this tree, like all trees, had its growth spurts where new branches and leaves and fruits appeared and had a period of dormancy when a pause was needed for new growth. And now in this season of ending the book, the tree, though winter, feels as if it is in full bloom and giving fruits, flowers, and shade to all those who will sit under it, and hopefully write as they do so.

We hope that those who read you, dear book, will be inspired to write, create, make art, dance, sing, write songs, play, improvise, become curious, and immerse in any creative activities that evoke paying more attention to the self. Writing magically can be done in one minute or one year, in a tiny apartment in the middle of an enormous urban city or alone on a mountaintop cabin in Montana or Katmandu, with deer walking by outside or in the destruction of war and with the hope of rebuilding. You, dear book, were written on computers, but some people may prefer or have to write with a pen or pencil, on paper: blank or lined with margins; some might trace words in the sand, or dust after an earthquake.

Thank you, book, for all of the gifts we have received, and that through publishing you we can share with others.

In gratitude,

Krystal and Tamar

Index